full of it

with love & light

xoxo,

Ellen

full of it

a story of
health &
Healing
to hell & back

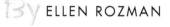 By ELLEN ROZMAN

Printed in the United States

First Printing, 2018

ISBN 978-0-9997439-0-4 (softcover)
ISBN 978-0-9997439-1-1 (hardcover)

Farm to Bedside Table Books

Cover design by Bianca Krause for The MOD Studio

Interior design by Marisa Jackson

Interior illustrations by Bianca Krause

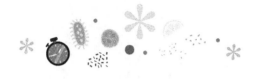

TO THE LOVES OF MY LIFE:

Mark, Harrison, and Shaine

For putting up with
all my Shit.

Table of Contents

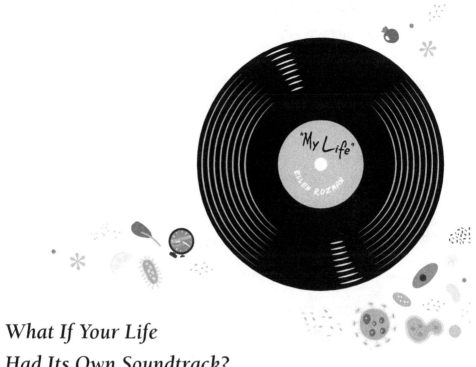

What If Your Life Had Its Own Soundtrack?

Music is magical. It's transformative, universal, cathartic. It takes us to places both familiar and unfamiliar, connects us to memories and creates new ones. It transcends age, gender, race, religion, and time. It's game-changing, mood-altering, and offers us the ultimate connection to one another. Music makes us move—dance, sing, cry. The tempo, the beat, the lyrics are expressions of our soul. The lyrics in the songs on the following pages resonated with me as I was writing these chapters. As you read through the chapters in this book, listen to the corresponding song on this Spotify list: http://bit.ly/fosbookplaylist. You can also create your own playlist and share it. It would be music to my ears to hear how your life has played out thus far.

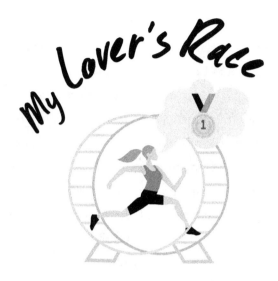

My Lover's Race

WHEN I FELL IN LOVE with exercise, I fell harder than I had for any human being. It's been the crux of my existence, the main source of my suffering, a hamster wheel that would not stop spinning. The affair began in high school when I ran distance on the cross-country team, prepping for my track season, and deepened during my gymnastic training in a school obsessed with success. The endorphins hooked me. My lover breathed down my neck, insisting I get faster, stronger, better, which silenced all thought, numbed all emotion, and eventually blinded me to the stranglehold this addiction had over my life.

When I left home to attend the University of Florida, my lover followed. I quickly connected with the girls in my sorority who were active in aerobics. Leg warmers and thong leotards were all the rage, and we couldn't get our neon-coated ass cracks out in public often enough. The Step craze was still in its infancy, but we loved bouncing up and down for hours, stepping on and off wooden boxes in rhythm to the music of Pat Benetar, Cindy Lauper, and Van Halen.

After college, when I moved to Birmingham to work as an assistant buyer at the upscale department store, Parisian, my lover moved too. We met again at my new gym, where we continued our devotion to Step classes. I loved our Step dates, so much so that when we missed one, I found myself riddled with anxiety, stress-filled, the world around me closing in on all sides. Attending classes kept me in check, balanced, and the music and choreography provided an outlet to escape my anxiety. Needless to say, we didn't miss many.

Soon I relocated to Atlanta to open Parisian's flagship store and manage the women's clothing department. My lover found me yet again, this time at a gym in Buckhead—one of the many gyms popping up all over the vast sprawling city—that had a huge aerobics room. My lover and I would join the line outside the door to sought-after-instructor Elaine's Step class, waiting in lusty anticipation, ready to move and sweat to the pumping beat of the music, high on the challenge of keeping up with the choreography of the class. We were so in love.

My lover kept our affair fresh by constantly morphing into something new that consumed me. Running was next. As a runner, my lover challenged my mind and my body. Reluctant at first (I really didn't like running), I agreed to train for a 10K run with some coworkers— The Peachtree Road Race in Atlanta, currently the largest 10K in the world (when I ran, there were a mere 50,000 runners). My lover tempted me as these friends promised it would be fun, nothing to worry about. We trained together after work in the evenings and occasionally on the weekends when we had time off.

Once again, I was hooked. My mindset was (as my lover knew it would be) if all those people could run it, I could too. But I was going to run the race on my own terms, so I set the bar at a time I considered acceptable (just above where I thought I'd be able to finish), but not out of reach. That way, I could prove to myself that I could do well even in my first timed race.

A few years later, on my first day living in Austin, not yet employed, I signed away a large part of my savings to a local gym, realizing my lover had followed me once again. But without much financial cushion, it never occurred to me that maybe my lover didn't always have my best interests at heart. Soon after moving to Austin, I started dating my future husband, Mark. I wondered how my new romance would go over with my lover, but it wasn't a problem. As long as I kept up our workouts, I was free to spend time with Mark as I desired. I balanced the two. I craved the time with my lover. At the gym. Running. I felt so energized. I had a desperate need to feel in control and my long, intense workouts fulfilled that need.

And I loved being with Mark. He was chill, calm, grounded, nonreactive, an energetic balance to my always running, moving, full of energy, boom, boom, go, go, go self. We explored the city together, hung out with friends, went to hear live music, ate out.

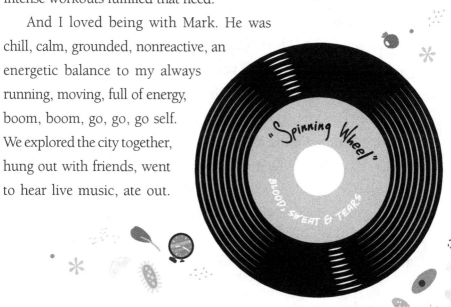

We both loved fitness, but different disciplines. Mark was a golfer and a swimmer, not a runner, which made me sad. By running together, he would see that I was strong and recognize my strength, ability, athleticism. I wanted to be complimented and acknowledged for a job well done. But that didn't happen. I didn't get what I was always striving for, that feeling of acceptance. So instead, my lover filled that need by providing me with feelings of self-worth and badassery from the events he lured me into, from those who were competing with me, and from others who recognized me as a fellow athlete and runner.

Several years later, now the mother of two, I overheard a conversation at the gym about a women's only triathlon. I was immediately intrigued—a new way to spend more time with my lover. For three months, my lover and I trained intensely, determined to complete this first triathlon. We got stronger, faster, and gained endurance. I entered one triathlon, then another, and another. I couldn't stop. I was always looking to improve my times.

Morphing once more, our affair became sweatier, more exhausting, more complex, and highly competitive. Our friendly competition was turning on me. I both loved and hated my lover, who fueled my greatest passion. I felt tugged in one direction while my heart strings pulled me in another, toward my family. I wanted Mark to allow me to put all my focus into my love affair with exercise, so, for my fortieth birthday, with more stamina than ever and the desire to complete a goal that was beyond my comfort zone, I asked Mark for a pretty huge gift—to help me prepare for the Wildflower Half Ironman distance triathlon, so I could once again one-up myself. I asked him to pick up our kids, Harrison and Shaine, from school when I was training with my group, to spend time with them on weekends while I was out on long rides or runs, to understand if I was too tired on the days I ran to cook dinner. He was torn, but he agreed.

As I trained, the guilt weighed heavy on my heart. Still, I wanted more—to get faster, stronger, to not only complete the race but to actually compete, to achieve an acceptable time, to finish in the top tier of my training group. I never stopped reaching. Constantly striving for more. Nothing could satisfy my desire to improve. The farther I went, the faster I became, the more I wanted—I just kept raising the bar. Higher and higher with no limits on how high I could take it. Each time I cranked my bike pedals, each time my foot left the pavement, I distanced myself further from my emotions, too far into the race to consider stopping.

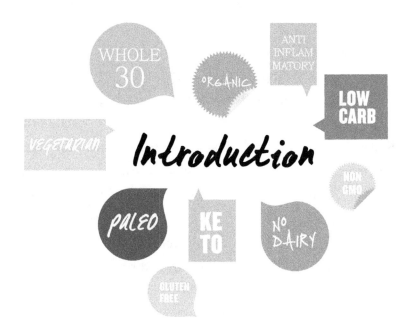

Introduction

WHAT I EXPERIENCED during much of my adult life is a condition that prevails in today's society and among women who are multi-tasking to the point of oblivion. We're moving in (or in my case, *running* in) circles and ending up further behind. We're obsessed with "stuff" and with accruing more of it, and we're trying to outpace our mortality, our sadness, our fears with whatever it is we don't have or haven't accomplished. Retail therapy is a thing. And women's book clubs are being replaced with GNOs (Girls Night Out), where wine flows faster than tears shed while reading a depressing novel. We look outside ourselves for the answers when they're right in front of us. They speak to us from our inner core. The only problem is that we won't slow down enough to listen. The external dialogue is so loud, we can't hear that tiny voice crying from within.

We all struggle with our inner demons and an unhealthy relationship with someone or something. Shit, if we didn't, we wouldn't be human. In my case, it was an addiction to exercise and an obsession with food. I'm not talking about your typical "see food" diet, but an obsession with the qualities of food. My obsession began by removing fatty foods from my diet, then animal proteins (except seafood), then foods that weren't clean in my opinion, and, finally, those that wrecked my digestion. I've always had an *infatuation* (pardon the pun) with food. I'm a believer in Hippocrates' saying, "Let food be thy medicine and medicine be thy food." That's always been the answer. My answer. The type, source, ingredients, and quality of food was the answer to all that ailed me, and my strong-willed nature and breadth of knowledge was my ultimate #fail.

I was also obsessed with doing too much, exercising too much, performing well, exceeding my self-imposed bar—all for the approval I craved, including my own, which was hard-won and short-lived. By the time I was in my early forties, I'd pushed myself so hard for so long—go, go, go—that I began to have serious issues with my gut (as in the literal form of go, go, go, read #2). I planned my long runs around available restrooms. I avoided parties, which I loved, because I knew I'd end up locked in the bathroom. I became depressed. I became a recluse, avoiding social interactions—parties, dinners, events—and activities with friends. I consulted doctors, nutritionists, gastroenter-ologists, acupuncturists, Ayurvedic practitioners, functional medicine docs, spiritual guides, energy healers, herbalists, an iridologist, even a Tarot card reader. I self-diagnosed, focusing closely, or solely, on my diet, studying which foods were "good to eat," and then determining which of those foods made my stomach bloated, gassy, and crampy.

I became interested in the source of my food and connected to the farmers who grew it. Nothing was clean enough. Every single thing I ate had to come from a source I knew. It had to be sustainable, local, whole, pure, free of dyes and chemicals. These were all symptoms of a condition known as orthorexia nervosa, where you start out eating healthfully, but eventually, food choices become so restrictive that your health suffers as a result.

I had cramps. My body ached because I didn't allow it to recover enough between runs. But I kept running anyway—first just four to seven miles, four days a week, 5Ks and 10Ks twice a month, and then half marathons (thirteen miles), which were somewhat manageable. Once I became more involved in the running community, the idea of running a marathon (which I'd said I would never do) became more appealing. *Not* because I enjoyed the distance running, but because it presented another challenge. And boy did it! The longer I ran during training runs, the worse I felt. But. I. Kept. Going. I completed three marathons (twenty-six miles) in my running career. I knew I should have stopped after the first, but as a goal-oriented, Type-A, driven idiot, I pushed. While that voice may have been shouting at me, I heard only a slight whisper, something I could easily drown out with my loud mind: *Just do it, you'll be fine. You did it yesterday and the day before, even though you felt the same way. You'll get too far behind. You'll lose your fitness. You're not a wimp. Just keep going.* Then there was the external chatter—the comments and questions from family and friends. And the physical cues—my weight loss, the constant bloat and gas I experienced.

Because my gut sometimes kept me from running as hard as I would have liked, being lean became especially important to me; the leaner I was, the faster I went. But I wasn't getting the nourishment I needed to fuel the amount of exercise I was doing. I wasn't getting enough nourishment, period. Equally, I grappled with my appearance. I had to look the part—triathlete, coach, trainer, group exercise instructor. There was (still is) a persona I felt pressured to fit. I lived in a continual struggle with my image issues, my performance issues, and I pressured myself to succeed in all my athletic endeavors, to hold onto my status as an athlete. I wanted to be who I imagined others thought I was, squashing the signs and symptoms that plagued my body as I continued to pound the pavement.

Some of my issues around food stemmed from being so hard on myself, not nourishing myself properly. I ate to feed my hunger, rather than nourish my body. It's not that I didn't appreciate food. I ate foods that felt safe to me, that wouldn't wreck my gut, at least on that given day, which meant that to satiate myself, I would eat and eat and eat, the same foods, and in large quantities. Now, years later, I appreciate food in a different way. I love to go out to eat and discover what chefs are doing with seasonal ingredients. Before, going out to eat was difficult because I was afraid to branch out too far from my comfort zone. I felt too nervous to experiment with new ingredients and new tastes.

Often, when I talk with friends, parents from my kids' school, others in the community, both moms and dads, the subject of food and exercise comes up. The conversation takes a predictable turn from the positive benefits of healthy eating and a moderate amount of exercise to a need (*read: addiction*), expectation (*of self or others*), requirement (*societal pressure*), or vanity (*I ate this so I have to exercise, I can't look a certain way, etc.*). We eat or don't eat for all kinds of reasons, but if you take a closer look, many of our food choices are made to fuel the expectations of ourselves or others—I'm a vegetarian. I'm vegan. I'm Paleo. I'm doing Whole30. I'm on a ketogenic diet.

Many of us also use food to punish or to reward ourselves, depending on what we think we deserve. Many of us love to exercise, but the absolute need to exercise can come when we let ourselves go, overindulge, or start to feel as though we "should" fit a certain mold or body type. When we force ourselves into believing that society's expectations of who we should be and how we should look are more important than our own—that's when we force ourselves into exercising to fit into our skinny jeans or favorite shorts from college. We start to believe it's no longer a choice. That's when we re-introduce the juice cleanse, the Whole30 diet, and renew our annual membership to the gym.

So as we consider our need or desire to exercise, we don't listen to our bodies when we feel off, have had a bad night's sleep, our allergies are acting up, or we've overdone it the day before. We push past what we innately feel and let our minds take over, forcing us to go to a place that contradicts our strongest internal signals. If we don't exercise, we'll fail.

We'll get behind (or get a big behind). And we'll lose everything we've worked for up to that point and have to start all over again. We'll feel like failures (so let's just fuckin' finish that pint of artisanal organic ice cream). We'll get sick (and then miss even more workouts). Other mind mantras might include: *My waist size will increase (read: bring skinny jeans to Goodwill). I'm not pretty, handsome, or fit (none of my friends or co-workers will want to include me in their #selfies). Everyone else is working out today (just insert big "L" on forehead for LOSER).* And on and on and on.

We do the same thing with food after we've gained a few pounds. We cleanse, restrict, punish—no matter what our gut tells us. It's signaling things like *Eat, dammit. I'm starving. Gimme meat. No more celery juice! Back off from dairy and citrus!* The problem is this: when we don't think we deserve much, we can't determine what's best for us. If we suffer from the feeling of not-enoughness, believing that we don't matter unless we are *achieving*, we're never going to feel we've done enough, are enough. We'll never win the race because the finish line keeps moving just out of reach.

As a health coach, my clients ask me what they should or should not eat to lose weight or become healthier. Initially, the conversation isn't about what's best for their specific, individual needs. Instead, they're looking beyond themselves to conform to cultural standards of beauty and they want to achieve that ideal weight or shape they see in ads or TV commercials. They might admire my physique, the fact that I'm thin, strong, and competitive. Many tell me up front that they *want* to be healthy, but they care too much about what they look like to consider how they're feeling (hungry, tired) as a deciding factor in how they take care of themselves. We work on that. I'm extremely qualified to work with those issues because I get it. I *totally* get it. I've been there.

I've struggled with similar issues for most of my life, feeling the pressure to fit a mold or conform to the perception of others rather than listening to, or even hearing, the cries of my inner voice and allowing myself to enjoy and express myself and my body as it is, or was. I'd shut off the volume to the internal signals originating from my gut, telling me what I needed, and instead force myself to stay the course. Whatever edible bandwagon I was currently on—no fat, only organic, no meat, whatever—I would not bend my rules. And nothing, no internal signals, no external signs, could steer me in another direction. I'm very headstrong, baby!

Once I became honest with myself and others about my struggles, my anxiety began to melt away. I could express myself without excuses or shame, be more present and authentic in all areas of my life. My hope is that the personal experiences I share in this book will inspire others struggling with this silent battle to tune into that voice in the depth of their core that's struggling to be heard. Or turn up the volume if necessary.

Many feel ashamed, embarrassed, or afraid to admit to their weaknesses. I might not be the first to tell you that fear is our biggest enemy, but I'm urging you to start working through it. Listen to those signs and signals from your heart, your spirit, and most important, your gut. Blast the knob to number 10. *All* those lyrics compose your song. The songs are singing your answers. If you can move toward facing those effing thoughts playing on the wrong frequency and quiet the static that surrounds them, you'll absolutely crush it and feel as though you've made it to the Top 40 chart. Even if you only achieve one-hit wonder status by acting on one thought, one feeling, one symptom—awesome! You'll still be a pop star in my book! Inspiring one another is what it means to be healthy, and I'm your Number One Fan!

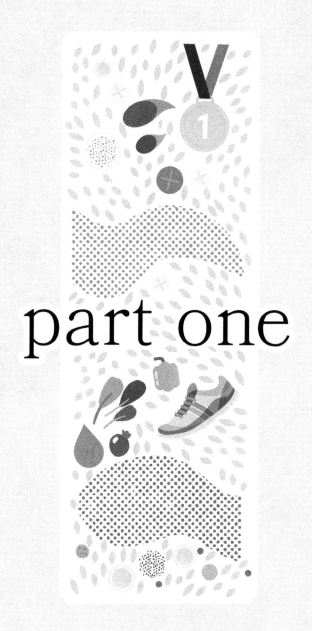

part one

Preaddict in Training

ALL MY LIFE I'VE WALKED the line between wanting to be different and wanting to be accepted, wanting to remain true to myself, but wanting others to value who I am. It's just that I couldn't stand still long enough to figure out who the hell that was. As a child, I remember being very focused on projects and performance—playing dodgeball, running relay races, and building sandcastles to the point of perfection—though my fierce independence didn't really take root until high school. Perhaps it was forged in my highly competitive private school in Uptown New Orleans. High school was tough for me, because even though I was extremely autonomous, I wanted to blend in with the girls in my class. That meant making a debut and going to the balls during Mardi Gras season. But, as a Jew in the '80s, I had to be asked as a date. I wasn't allowed to make a debut or participate in the queens' court, as so many girls from my school did. No matter how much effort I put into being accepted, I would still lack the credentials needed to be welcomed into the inner circle of New Orleans, and the festival that is so much a part of my hometown.

Many of my friends and peers were active debutantes, and around Mardi Gras season, they'd attend events, balls, and dinners. The krewes—the exclusive groups who host the Mardi Gras balls and events—would elect these debs to a place on the queen's court or, in certain cases, as queen of that particular krewe, which was a tremendous honor and the highest status among those in the inner circle.

Throughout high school, I attended a handful of the balls as the date of various boys in my class. The guys whose families were affiliated with the krewes had no restrictions on whom they could bring. Luckily, for me, this was a way in. I was well liked enough to get asked by some of my guy friends as their date and was able to party with the best of 'em!

The experience was certainly one to be remembered. The formality of it seemed odd to me, yet it was also enticing and curious, and the parties after the balls were like nothing I'd ever experienced. The venues were huge and beautifully decorated. There was a formal presentation of the court where people paraded around in their finest ball gowns, food stations galore, and dancing and drinking and more drinking. This ended before midnight, then the Queen's supper began. That's when the party really started. I remember getting home after 2:00 a.m. (and that was an early curfew), but those parties lasted into the wee hours, sometimes until 4:00 a.m. My inclusion in this generations-old tradition masked my feelings of being an outsider, different and not accepted.

One organization, in particular, operated a bit differently from the rest. They invited Jews to participate in the company of the court. Jews weren't asked to be on the court—just in the company. Like, sit on the floor and watch everyone else walk by in their floor-length gowns with their scepters and crowns kind of included. Still, it was my ticket inside, and when I received my invitation, I was totally on board! The fifty to seventy-five girls each paying a $250 fee to take part were given pastel clown costumes to wear at the ball. During my freshman and sophomore years, I happily obliged. It was fun while it lasted, and then, one day, the foolishness of it all set in.

In the fall of my junior year, when once again the invitation arrived in the mail, I opened it in disgust and said to myself, *Why would I pay $250 to sit my ass on the floor and dress like a clown?* I ripped up the invitation, and, after that, I stopped caring about having anything to do with the balls. I could feel a change inside me. I'd spent a good many years being worried about peer acceptance, and then that day I thought, *This is crazy!* I wasn't going to clown around anymore.

The joke was on them! I was rebelling against what I knew was unjust and humiliating. I was beginning to discover my true self, and what mattered to me most at that time was a sense of realness.

Standing up for myself in an adolescent, awkward, and isolated space was scary, though I was starting to get in touch with who I really was and what made me tick. I realized being authentic and loyal to my feelings was better than masquerading behind something that I thought would make me feel more connected, but, in reality, made me feel more like an outsider—able to peek in from the windows but not allowed to enter through the door.

Still, this realization remained only a whisper as I channeled that need to fit in and excel into school. My high school was a small and exclusive environment filled with competitive, smart, talented kids who were driven to be better, faster, smarter—to get the award, to win the race. I fit right in. In addition to academics, it focused on participation in athletics, student government, school clubs, and philanthropy.

I joined Booster Club, Philanthropic Committee, French Club. I volunteered as a candy striper in a local hospital and for the annual telethon at the local PBS station. I ran for and was elected to senior class something (Secretary? Treasurer? I can't remember). I made cheerleader—a sought-after and high-profile position at my school. I was on the Homecoming Court, which was voted on by the senior class. I had a single-minded determination. If I wanted something bad enough, I went after it. And I got it—well, most of the time. But all through those years, I ran the never-ending dialogue in my head, comparing myself with my classmates—making sure I was doing "just as much" as they were.

And while the pressure I put on myself in my social and academic life was pretty intense, that pressure was nothing compared with how I handled my athletic endeavors.

In the spring of my freshman year, I went out for the track team, running the 400-meter dash. While I performed somewhere in the middle of the pack—I was a good athlete but not the greatest—my drive and determination worked to improve my ranking. I loved the feeling of accomplishment at the end of a race. Each time I saw my splits, I would strive to one-up myself. I ran cross country to help improve my times and gain endurance and strength for the track season. Every day after school, for hours—around the track, along the levees, pounding the pavement and the neutral ground between the streetcar tracks up and down the avenues surrounding my school.

Running to the point of nausea. By the time I'd get home, I'd be too exhausted to eat dinner and wanted nothing more than to lie down and sleep. My body was totally spent. My periods were all screwed up—they'd stop and start, then stop again. Not exactly regular for a fifteen-year-old. When my weight dropped, my mother became alarmed and eventually, after a dramatic office visit to an endocrinologist, I was forced to stop running. No negotiation. I was really pissed. I certainly didn't love running, but it had become part of my identity.

Quitting, especially at my school, at my age, and with my mentality was not an option. It would make me look bad. It would mean I wasn't good enough, that I was backing down and couldn't handle the pressure or intensity. I felt as though I had something to prove to myself and others, that I was competitive, an athlete, and that I could perform. Still, running was out. So the Monday following my doctor's appointment, after I had a complete meltdown over the weekend about not being able to continue my running, I tried out for the gymnastics team, and I made it.

At that time, in the very early '80s, no one realized how intense and fiercely competitive the sport was, or my parents (and probably my doctors) wouldn't have let me try out. The sport was dominated by women from the Soviet Union and Eastern Europe.

"Can't Stop This Feeling"

JUSTIN TIMBERLAKE

The foreign elite gymnasts (Nadia Comǎneci and Olga Korbut) were petite, very lean, and flexible. It wasn't until the 1984 Olympics that Mary Lou Retton, a US power gymnast, proved the petite but muscular and thicker body type could produce the same, if not more, impressive results. After that, the sport went in a different direction. The tricks became much tougher to perform, requiring more power and strength from increased muscle mass.

But when I was on the team, the lighter and leaner, the better— the higher you could fly. All this pressure on body type and weight created a "secret society" of many up-and-coming gymnasts obsessed with food and rooted in the need to maintain an extremely challenging size. No one really discussed this, but the gymnasts all knew about it. And the coaches were the ones driving the train.

The practices were long and arduous, and once I began practicing and competing with the team, I realized how intense the sport was— but I never admitted this to my parents. They would have made me quit. And I did not want to quit. Gymnastics allowed me to cling to that intensity I craved, a way for me to express my athleticism, strength, competitive nature, and my desire to succeed.

I was already thin, though I didn't exactly have the petite frame of a gymnast. I was 5'7", averaging three to five inches taller than most of my teammates. But the lighter I became, the better advantage I had. I'd always been interested in food and nutrition, but to stay leaner, I became even more so. I started reading everything I could on the subject. I was like a sponge. I poured over *Mademoiselle*, *Glamour*, and *Seventeen* for their articles about which foods were healthiest. I became more conscious of what I ate. While I was not anorexic—I ate a lot—I was very selective about what I'd eat.

Back then, calories were all about count, not content. It's completely the opposite these days. Crystal Light was new on the scene, and I made pitchers of the lemonade, day after day after day. I crunched on celery and carrot sticks with low-fat Hidden Valley Ranch dressing, consumed lots of carbs, a little protein, and absolutely no fat—those were the days of, "Fat is bad. Fat makes you fat." Anything considered low or no-fat passed inspection in my book. I had no regard for the quality of ingredients. Homing in on the calorie and fat content on the nutrition label was my only concern—a diet mentality that likely set my gut up for what was to come.

I developed body-image issues; probably, in part, because what I put in my mouth I could control, and I wanted control. I maintained this façade of control with a combination of exercise and food. I was obsessed with being the best I could be, and my secret weapon was my nutrition. I dialed in to what all the magazines told me I should do to become "healthier" and "fitter." I wanted to look the part and knew that my lighter frame would allow me to bend, twist, and fly more easily, so keeping my weight down became a priority.

And I lost who I was, or, really, who I was becoming. In high school, many girls, just like me, were trying to figure out who they were too, overachieving to be recognized. We were all trying to stand out and blend in at the same time, assert our independence while still being accepted by others.

My food, my athletics, my involvement in activities—both in school and out—were the costume for those emotions. A way to disguise what I was feeling inside. But in spite of my finest accomplishments, these perceptions paraded on. So I continued to satiate my emotional hunger with empty calories, until, eventually, that feeling

I'd tried to repress—of never being good enough or doing enough —came back to bite me in the ass.

Harder, Better, Faster, Stronger

MY NEED TO PROVE MYSELF grew stronger every year and continued into my adult life. Once I felt I'd reached a certain level of achievement, I was determined to exceed it. If I was the chair of a fundraiser, I had to surpass the fundraising goal. And if I was asked to chair it again, I would need to outperform myself by exceeding the previous year's gross. After I threw my two-year-old daughter a magical princess birthday party, I had to get more creative about the cake, the theme, the favors for her third birthday. Each year my holiday Sip and Shop had to be more elaborate than the previous year's—more vendors, more food, more people, longer days.

I was often complimented on my ability to put on an event, chair a fundraiser, throw a party. I thrived on the positive feedback, never slowing down to wonder why I needed it so much. "How do you do it all, and so well?" my friends asked. I didn't realize it at the time, but my body was paying the price for my inability to slow down—

my gut was slightly off, but I thought it was the norm. I was busy! Always busy, constantly busy. Then there were all the moms I compared myself to, moms who worked and attended board meetings and volunteered. *If they can do it, I can do it*, I told myself. It didn't matter what it was—volunteering, completing a triathlon, improving my times, being more involved in my kids' schools, whatever—I tackled it.

It was as though someone had programmed that Kanye West song "Stronger" in my head, and had it set on a never-ending loop: "Harder, better, faster, stronger. . . ." If I didn't continue to do better, do more, to improve beyond my own benchmark and outperform myself, I felt worthless. The voice in my head never stopped asking "Why?" *Why shouldn't I be able to keep all the balls in the air when I've done this for so long?* Then there were those who were concerned I was doing too much, like Mark and my parents. And people who were constantly commenting on my involvement in so many activities, which caused me to wonder, *Why is everyone questioning why I have to take on this task? Why, when there are so many other women who work full-time jobs, have kids, and do tons of volunteer work, am I being singled out as the one who's doing too much?*

Exercise was the one area where I found release. While I pushed myself hard—teaching spinning classes every Wednesday for years, spending every spare moment I could at the gym—I had a tough time taking days off. I felt an energetic connection to the space and the people. I also felt like I would fall behind if I didn't exercise. I'd lose my strength. I'd be impossible to live with. It was my release, my vice, something I had to accomplish to feel complete. It was my way to get "the wiggles out," to release the stressors of everyday life, to focus on a goal—running a certain distance, achieving five hundred steps on the elliptical, feeling my body heat and heart rate increase. While I had always craved exercise, I was also attracted to the community and the enjoyment of the high-intensity group sweat sessions. Even my running—the 5Ks and 10Ks I sporadically entered—was socially focused, and I entered these races more for the love of community, intensity, and accomplishment than for the love of competition.

I developed a social circle at my gym—I was there all the time, for long periods of time. I saw the same group of people every day. Instead of talking "gym smack" all the time, we began to share more personal stories with one another, whether they were work-related, relationship-related, kid-related, whatever. We formed a bond, a tight bond. We didn't compete with each other. But that all changed when I hit my early thirties, and some friends talked me into entering a triathlon. Once the triathlon bug bit, my mindset shifted. Everything kicked up a notch. The competitive drive grabbed me. Nothing, nothing, nothing hooked me the way triathlons did. Triathlons fueled the drive to outdo myself, that sense of one-upping myself each and every time I raced. I was always looking at my times and holding myself accountable to be "better, faster, stronger" each race, each year. Although I continued to chair events, put on fundraisers, and sit on numerous boards, nothing made me feel more complete than training for and competing in triathlons.

A triathlon has three parts, or splits. You typically start off with an open water swim, followed by the bike portion, and ending with a run, with a transition between each sport. The swim-to-bike transition is called T1. The bike-to-run transition is T2. Back when I was racing, our times were captured by chips strapped to our ankles. That's old school now (shows you how old I am!). There are generally four triathlon distances: Sprint, Olympic, Half Ironman, and Ironman. For my first tri, I decided to enter a sprint, which is composed of a half-mile swim, a bike portion ranging from twelve to fifteen miles, and a 5K run (3.1 miles)—about one-quarter of a Half Ironman and one-eighth of a full one. It was an all-women's triathlon called the Danskin, which took place in several cities around the United States. I competed in the Austin race. I borrowed a bike from a friend and trained with her for two to three months before the event.

In the week preceding that first race I felt stressed out and nervous, but when all was said and done, my time turned out okay. So when I finished, I thought, *Now that I've got one in the books, I know I will be able to do so much better next time!* And so it began. I entered another. And another. And another. For seven years, from January through June, I was training—running, biking, and swimming. And from June through August I was either training or racing. I loved training. I loved the challenge, the feeling of exhaustion, the sense of accomplishment. I could barely handle the triathlons themselves—I hated the stress—but I had to race. I needed that sense of self-worth that came from crossing the finish line. I competed in the same races, on the same courses every year and each time I raced, I expected to improve my times. I was always checking my splits: *What time do I have to beat for my swim? What time do I have to beat for my bike? My run? How fast do I need to be in my transitions?* Ad nauseum.

I entered more than forty triathlons, graduating from Sprint to Olympic. My kids were in grade school then, and I often missed after-school or weekend swim meets, soccer games, and baseball games because I was training or racing. Sometimes I would arrive late because I'd been out in the middle of nowhere Texas on a long ride and I couldn't get back in time.

Other times I was doing bike/run bricks, where I'd bike long and hard enough to get my legs fatigued and then hop off the bike for a run. Your legs feel like bricks (hence the term) as your feet shuffle along the pavement during the transition from peddling to running. As much as I wanted to be at my kids' games and meets, as guilty as I felt about not being there, the drive to train so that I would perform well won out every time. It was my exercise addiction talking, my urge to compete. I couldn't think rationally.

Knowing my kids had a sporting event made me run harder, pedal faster. I constantly checked my watch for my time, calculating how many more miles I had to pedal before I got back to the car to battle traffic and dash in for the last inning of the baseball game or the final event in the swim meet. I always showed up with a tremendous feeling of guilt. I wondered what the other moms and dads thought as I came racing in, a sweaty stinkin' mess, with helmet head and grease marks on my calves from my bike chain. I don't think the kids knew how much of their games and swim meets I missed. I just know they were happy to see me there.

Mark was supportive. He knew this was my thing. But after a few years, my weekend schedule was creating stress for the whole family. I felt guilty and torn. I missed my kids. I missed Mark. They missed me. And as much as Mark enjoyed spending time with the kids during the weekends, he needed some downtime from his work week. It was asking a lot of him to bear the brunt of weekend childcare. What was worse, in the weeks before a race, I was physically and emotionally unavailable. I'd put an incredible amount of pressure on myself, becoming highly stressed. I could feel everything around me start to close in. I was short with Mark and really quiet, really into myself, because that's how I get when I'm stressed, I'm just like, "Don't talk to me, don't mess with me, I'm on a mission." But once I committed to a race, I *had* to follow through with results.

I would completely focus on the race, and as it drew closer my head was constantly spinning with the minutiae of the event: *What is the weather going to be like? Should I bring an extra towel? Should I wear socks?* (Putting socks on took 2.5 seconds with my feet a little wet and muddy from running up from the lake.) My thoughts were filled with little details: What to pack, how I would improve my times, who was competing in my age group, what food I should bring. I'd visualize the course—would it be wet, dry, muddy, cold? Would the hills slow me down? What was the elevation on the run course? The more these worries filled my head, the less I wanted to interact with anyone else. I was completely immersed in thoughts about how I would perform.

I kept at it, and when my fortieth birthday was a little more than six months away, I was training and competing with more stamina and determination than I'd had in my entire life. I decided to enter a Half Ironman. I know a lot of people take a trip for milestone birthdays. They throw big parties, go out and get shit-faced to both celebrate and drown their sorrows about getting older. Crap, several women I know got boob jobs. Not me. No way. Small boobs were the ticket if you wanted to run fast. You just smushed them in a sports bra and that was it. No doubling up. Many women wear two sports bras to "hold it all in" so they don't bounce all over the run course. Not me. No chafing under the arms. It was awesome!

I wanted to give myself the gift of entering a Half Ironman. Not a full Ironman. I just didn't enjoy running enough, and I realized how daunting it would be and how my body would totally reject running a full marathon after swimming 2.5 miles and biking 112. I knew inside that it was much more than I could handle, both physically and emotionally.

Triathlon results are shown by age group. In some of the Sprint or Olympic distance triathlons I used to compete in, I might rank in the top ten overall in my age group. In the swim and bike, my times could hover in the top ten, though my run times usually placed me somewhere between twelve and twenty. Running twenty-six miles after swimming and biking would just be too taxing on my system. But I knew I could do a Half Ironman. I could give that to myself. And from Mark, I wanted the gift of time—six months to train specifically for a Half Ironman distance tri. Before I presented my plan to him, I wanted to get all my details in place. I went online, searching for destination races, and found one, the Wildflower triathlon at Lake San Antonio in central California.

This race is the Woodstock of the Half Ironmans. Very granola-ish. All the participants pitch tents at the surrounding campground. The Grateful Dead plays in the background during training runs and the subtle yet prevalent smell of weed fills the clean California air. One of the local colleges always hosts a water stop along the run course— college kids handing you water with a splash of T & A. At that point, you're kind of delusional, but the fact that they're passing out water and Gatorade in the nude is definitely something that puts a smile on your face! The lake temp is a chilly 65 degrees, the bike course is very hilly. Overall, Wildflower is a tough race.

I'm not some Jewish American Princess, but I'm not all that rustic either. Actually, I am not rustic at all. I like hiking and being outdoors, but camping has never been my vibe. I'm not into building a fire, cooking dinner in the coals, zipping myself into a sleeping bag at the end of the day. This place went so completely and totally against my grain, but it was supposed to be a really, really fun experience. I thought, *Why not? I'm turning forty! I'm going to go totally outside my box.*

I not only wanted the gift of time from Mark, I really wanted him to come with me, to share in the experience. I wanted his full support. I told him I'd fly out with the team, do some training on the course, and get settled in. He could meet up with me the day before and watch the race. Then we could leave the campsite and drive up the coast to Carmel and Big Sur to relax, unwind, and celebrate. It would be the perfect little vacation, providing us with some quality time together after six long months of training. It was a great plan. It took some convincing, but he grudgingly agreed. I was thrilled.

I joined the Leukemia & Lymphoma Society's Team in Training program. They sponsor triathlons, marathons, 5Ks, bike rides, and other athletic endeavors. They provide the coaches, connect you with a team, and cover your entry fee and part of your expenses. In turn, you fundraise. I had to raise about $4,000 to participate in Wildflower.

I sent an email to friends, family, and clients explaining that in lieu of throwing a big party for the Big 4-0, I wanted to do something for me, but I also wanted to give back while doing it. This was the best of both worlds. I happily and easily accomplished my fundraising goal.

I started training with my LLS team. Most of the participants in the group I trained with were younger than I was, only a handful were married, and I was one of only two moms. Neither of us had full-time jobs. The group trained on the weekends, and occasionally, though very rarely, I joined them for the evening workouts during the week. Four days a week, I'd teach a spin class or workout in the mornings, maybe fit in a personal training session with a client, and then head back to the Jewish Community Center at noon for a masters swim workout. I also joined a running group. I figured since running was my weakest area, to improve my age-group ranking and overall time, I had to really focus my efforts there. So, in addition to my LLS team workouts, I started working with a running coach, Cassie.

I sometimes pushed myself so hard when swimming or running that I hated every minute of it. Often, if not always, I had butterflies in my stomach before a challenging workout, knowing that I was about to suffer. I was mentally fighting a battle each and every time I stepped onto the pavement or suited up for a swim. (The bike was not as much of a mental struggle for me. It wasn't quite as intense or claustrophobic.) This was the beginning of my gut really acting up when I ran long distances. On the weekends, when I ran with my friend Noel, just as I approached the seven-mile mark, my belly began to feel like it was going to explode, and I'd have to stop running. Completely stop, and dart into the nearest fast food restaurant, grocery store, gas station—wherever I could find a bathroom. My belly also revolted during my running group workouts, but because the group met for only an hour, I'd usually make it through. But when I got home, my insides would just come out of me. I'd run into the bathroom and explode. It was horrible.

When I told my LLS coach about my bowel problems, he suggested eliminating gluten. This was before being GF was a thing. I talked with a nutritionist, who said it would take about six weeks to eliminate gluten from my system, so I stopped eating it right away. From that moment forward I made absolutely certain to only eat foods that were gluten-free (and it wasn't easy then—nothing was labeled). I had eight weeks until Wildflower and would do anything to make sure I didn't cramp up or have to poop during that race. It would certainly take too much time—I had to meet my time goal!

Two nights before the race, I flew out with my team, loaded down with all my clothes for the swim, bike, and run. I packed my wetsuit, running shoes, bike shoes, socks, race belt, and towel for my transition area. I filled a Ziploc with GU Energy Gel and Hammer Gel for fuel and another with snacks to eat in the tent. Since we were camping, I borrowed a headlamp, a sleeping bag, and a tarp to put under my sleeping bag in case the ground was wet. I took sweats and heavy socks to sleep in, and multiple changes of clothes for racing and training. Plus toiletries, underwear, towels, and flip-flops for the showers.

We landed in Oakland, piled into shuttles, and drove an hour south to Lake San Antonio, where we spent two nights at the campsite. The first night I was in the tent solo. The second night, the night before the race, Mark flew in and stayed with me in the tent. I didn't sleep at all. The ground was uneven. It was noisy, a total festival atmosphere. People were partying and smoking in the campsite right next to us. It was chilly—high 50s, low 60s—and I don't tolerate the cold well. My toes were numb, and when my feet are cold, I can't sleep. I got up to pee three times in the middle of the night because I'd drunk so much fluid out of fear that I would bonk the next day. Each time, I had to locate the damn headlamp so I could find my way. Then I had to find my hiking boots or tennis shoes so I could maneuver to the restroom—a cinderblock square building with multiple stalls and sinks, with that over-sanitized campsite restroom smell and too many glaring fluorescent lights. I'd wait in line for a stall, pee, wash my hands in the rust-stained sink, wipe them on my sweats, and stumble back to my tent to try and get some shut eye before I woke up to pee again. Glamping this was not.

All I have to do is think about Wildflower, and it's like I'm right there. In the midst of it. The images are so sharp in my mind. As though it's happening at this moment. This is how I recall it playing out . . .

The Swim: I have no idea about the current. How rough it might be. We start out in waves, by age group. Three to five minutes between each wave. Starting out is the worst. The freezing water. The crush of bodies. Two hundred swimmers elbowing, kicking to claim their space. I'm swimming for dear life—to beat my time, to break free of the pack, to outswim that sense of panic I get almost every time I jump in the water. Think butterflies, nausea, and nervousness that you're going to drown and get trampled—all tangled in one large knot in your gut. Add in a good kick or elbow in the side, and you are on the verge of puking. It gets better after that. You just have to pull away from the pack and find your own space to swim. Kick, pull, kick, pull, kick harder.

T1. Back on land. I check my watch to see my swim split. I rip off my wetsuit, dry off, pull on my socks and bike shoes. I grab my helmet, make my way to my bike, get myself out of the transition zone, mount my bike, and ride, ride, ride. The Bike: This is where I feel the most confident, secure. So free. Fifty-six miles through the rolling California hills. Beautiful terrain—wild grasses, scrub oaks, ponderosa pines—but I don't pay much attention. I'm uberfocused on the device on my handlebars that's constantly giving me feedback on my watts (how much power I'm putting out), RPMs (cadence), and speed. When I'm not checking the computer, I'm focusing on the bikes around me and the ground, watching for potholes or broken glass. I'm missing out on all the natural beauty and unfamiliar territory I'm weaving through.

As a team, we drove and rode the bike course the previous day. I know what to expect. I know where the hills are, the fast downhills that I can take advantage of to help improve my time. Toward the beginning there's an arduous one-mile grind. Brutal. All the way up, I keep telling myself that if I did it once, I can do it again. No way, no how will I get off my bike and walk it uphill. Not acceptable. If anyone else wants to do it, that's one thing. But it's absolutely not okay if I do. No more huge hills until the end of the ride, where there's this big ass hill called Nasty Grade. It's nearly five miles, 1,000 feet. I'll never forget that last climb. My quads on fire, I'm standing up on my pedals, grunting with all my might to make it to the top. I see people alongside me suffering too, some walking, though most grit their teeth and bear it just like me. If we have any amount of extra energy or breath, we cheer each other on, saying, "Great job" and "You got this." It's that little bit of encouragement that gets us through. Then we're at the finish.

T2. Check my watch, jump off my bike, run my bike to the transition line, rack my bike, swap out shoes, grab a hat, more GU, hydration, and run, run, run.

The Run: Focus, Ellen, focus! I'm struggling. The relentless push-push-push. I can't let up, I won't let up. I'm so fatigued from cranking circles for so long, and from that nasty final climb. My quads, filled with lactic acid—think jelly legs—barely able to put one foot in front of the other, but the adrenaline keeps me on track and focused, determined to finish this last leg of the race. My toes are stuck together from the hard-soled bike shoes. My heart is still beating a mile a minute from the last climb on the bike course, quickly getting into and out of the transition area, starting off on my run . . . I'm totally stressing myself out. There's so much yammering in my head: *I'm on the last leg. I can do this. I have to move quickly. Stay strong and run FAST to beat my goal time and beat the women in my age group.* I know when I want to finish and what time I need on my splits to make that happen. *No glory, all guts.* No time to enjoy the scenery, energy, and festivity surrounding me. I'm too serious. It's all a head game. I just want to finish with an acceptable time, for me, and we all know what "acceptable" means in my vocabulary. For anyone else doing this for the first time, especially a Half Ironman, especially Wildflower, the goal was to finish! But I had a single-minded focus. My eyes were on the woman wearing the red shorts about fifty feet in front of me. She was in my wave (our start order in the race, by age group), and I could tell by the number written in black Sharpie on the back of her calf (her age). *Get her. Pass her. Beat her.* I kept hearing in a loop in my head.

And then, unbelievably, I'm crossing the finish line. The experience is orgasmic—as good as sex. Every time. The high, the feeling of vulnerability, euphoria, the sense of accomplishment, the knowledge that my body is more powerful than my mind, the sweat on my bare skin, the amazing feeling that lasts for a day, maybe three . . . until I start training for my next race. But what I don't know is that this is my last triathlon.

The next few days were spent in a beautiful resort in Big Sur, on the California coast, the complete antithesis of the accommodations I'd tolerated those nights prior to Wildflower. The soft cotton sheets, the warm shower, the salt water pool, the organic food (including home-made granola each morning). It was all glorious. Mark and I walked along the beach, sat by the pool, drank wine, explored the nearby towns, and relaxed in the cool ocean air. It was a wonderful way to decompress after the duress I had put my body and mind through while preparing for Wildflower.

After nearly eight years, Mark was totally done with me and my training regimen. And for all those years, I'd been torn up inside about spending so much time away from my family and being so, well, pos-sessed. It was clear I had to make a change. My family, myself included, had had enough. When I mentioned to a few friends that I was con-templating a change, they suggested I race for fun. "Just go back and race sprints like you used to. You wouldn't even have to train. Just do them for fun," they would say. "My brain doesn't work that way," I told them. I couldn't race to have fun! I raced to improve. It was clear. To me, this was not a recreational sport. It was an expression of my ath-leticism and I took it seriously. If I quit, I had to quit cold turkey. And that's exactly what I did.

While my triathlon days were over, the drive to compete was not. Harder, better, faster, stronger ruled my every move—all this drive, and nowhere to put it. So, revved on high, I searched for another outlet.

Running with Moms

AFTER I QUIT triathlons, I transferred my entire focus to running. Every Sunday morning, I ran with my friend Noel. During the week, I did a few runs myself and on Wednesday mornings, from 9:15 to 10:15, I ran with the group of women runners I'd joined while training for the Wildflower triathlon. When I'd first considered joining the group, I was hesitant. These women ran 5Ks, 10Ks, half-marathons (13.1 miles), and marathons (26.2 miles). I'd only run a handful of 5Ks and 10Ks, with no desire to run more. I hated running. To me, it was just pounding and panting and more pounding. I wasn't one of those runners who took time to appreciate the scenery on my route—the color of a front door, an interesting landscape design, a new restaurant— I ran to get it done. But something felt different about how I approached running on those mornings with my running group. Instead of running *away from* something, whether it was self-judgment, fear, stress, uncertainty, I'd found a space where I could run *with*. With real, true, authentic human beings. A happy place that involved building friend-ships, connections, sharing, authenticity, encouragement, comfort, joy, and power.

Apart from all being moms, we couldn't have been more differ-ent. In the beginning, I was a triathlete whose least favorite sport was running, and I was only running with the group to improve my time in the Wildflower triathlon. They ran because they loved it. I lived in a different neighborhood. I was Jewish. Many belonged to the same church and attended a women's Bible study group together after our Wednesday runs. Their kids went to the same school. They hung out together. Their families hung out together. These women had been friends for years. Best friends. Even more than that, they were like soul sisters. But never in my life had I felt so accepted by and so close with a group of women.

From the very first day they welcomed me as one of their own. No questions asked. They didn't know who I was, where I lived, my reli-gion, what brand of running tights I had on—I could have been some snobby bitch from the other side of town. They didn't care; they just said, "We're so happy that you're a part of us." These women embraced me. One time I apologized—I think it was for being late—and I got called out: "We don't apologize here. You didn't do anything wrong. We're all human. We support each other."

That was so strange for me to hear, because it was so different from what my inner critic was constantly telling me—that I needed to be superhuman. I needed to exceed their expectations. As the new kid on the track, I needed to prove myself—my worth, my speed, my friendship. I wanted to do everything right for fear of being judged about something they wouldn't like or that they frowned upon. Little did I realize when I joined them that judgment, criticism, cattiness, and gossip were not a part of their vocabulary or existence. All the thoughts about how I should be, what I should say, or how I should look didn't apply when I was with them.

In my experience, the kind of acceptance and inclusion they showed me is rare. These women had such clarity about who they were. And because of that, to them, it had nothing to do with what was on the outside—they couldn't have cared less if I had a huge zit on my forehead or my eyebrows needed waxing. They cared about what was on the inside, which, for me, was a type of acceptance I'd never felt to that degree. All my life, with women who weren't my close friends, and sometimes with those who were, I'd always felt I had to prove—on the outside—that I was worthy of acceptance. I had to earn it. Overachieve. Fit into the mold I thought they had carved for me. So I pushed myself to perform beyond a level that I assumed others expected of me.

But when I met this group, I went in completely vulnerable. I had no idea how to dress, yet they could have cared less if I had Lulu or lint on my ass. They weren't making any judgments from my outward appearance. I wasn't going to blow their socks off with my running either. And they didn't care.

It was about encouragement. Those who finished first—always the same women—encouraged the others. They were always cheering on the rest of the group—clapping, wooing, and hooing at the top of their lungs. So thrilled that we finished, that we pushed hard, and so excited to give us those sweaty hugs and high fives as we crossed the finish line. They might have been more excited than we were in those moments. The approach was always, "We're in it together and we're here to support each other." That was it. It was just an incredible experience, making the intensity of the workouts worth every gasp of breath, every drop of sweat.

During this time, my tummy troubles continued and worsened. I began self-diagnosing (something I did a lot then) to determine what foods were affecting my gut, and slowly began eliminating them. I'd suspect something was contributing to the uncomfortable symptoms and soon enough, it was off the list of what I could eat: *Can't eat citrus anymore. It causes cramping. Can't eat raw cruciferous vegetables (cauliflower, broccoli, cabbage, etc.) either. They cause bloating and give me gas. Definitely not fatty fish. It bloats me and gives me diarrhea.* It was all supposition on my part, all an attempt to get to the "root cause" of my issue.

I never connected the dots—that my running was a contributing factor to my tummy troubles. It simply never occurred to me. Maybe because it was so important to me to maintain a strong, healthy, thin, muscular physique, and to do that, I kept pushing myself, while simultaneously eliminating foods from my diet. The list of what I felt I couldn't eat grew and grew, adding to the list of what I just didn't eat, which I conflated with who I was. I didn't eat red meat or poultry, and fish only occasionally, because, for the most part, I identified as a vegetarian. That was one of my labels. Part of my identity. I didn't eat dairy or gluten because neither really agreed with my digestion.

Finally, after about two years, I was left with a handful of foods that didn't dramatically affect my tummy. My daily diet was pretty much rice cakes (at least one sleeve per day if not more, often with almond butter), a banana, my signature trail mix (lots and lots of nuts, dried berries, and cacao nibs I'd put in snack bags and take wherever I went), goji berries, apples (with almond butter), and raw veggies like carrots and celery sticks (which I later discovered were a big contributing factor to my tummy troubles). I was always tired. And no wonder. On that diet, I was not getting enough nutrients.

Still, I kept running, and getting thinner. I not only wanted to run to improve, but I needed the running group, that particular group of women. For many reasons, some of which to this day I can't express in words. I sought their support, affirmation, and encouragement more than anything else. They always made me feel I was better than I thought I was—a better runner, friend, mom, wife, volunteer. They were there to show me I was "good enough," even though my mind was constantly telling me to do better. During the three years we trained together, many of the women would have to skip a Wednesday workout for whatever reason—meetings, school commitments, personal commitments, travel. Some would even stop coming for weeks or maybe a few months just to take a break from the intensity. But I never did. Not once. I couldn't stand missing a Wednesday morning and my weekly connection to these women. If it was pouring rain, I'd go. Freezing cold, yep, I'd be there too.

On those cold, wet days, often only three of us would show up. No matter how much I hated the cold, no matter how much I hated feeling all stuck together with sweat and rain, driving home soaked and shivering, it didn't matter. I went. It was the delight in sharing the experience with women who would say in between breaths, "I just love running in the rain!" and "This is so much fun!" Drenched shoes and all. It was a magical bond I'd formed—real women, real people, real friends. How could I have been surrounded by so many friends all my life and not known how beautifully supportive women could be? This group of women I had not previously known were the women who saved my life.

I believe now that the Universe brought them to me to establish trust so I could begin to see that I was more than my outward appearance, that I was substantial and had something I could pass on to others. They supported each other through loss and sorrow, through celebration and joy. And I was part of that. If they called me out on my behavior, my weight, my appearance, I tried to listen. Unfortunately, though, trying wasn't good enough here. I had much more suffering to endure before I chose to actually hear what they had to say.

Are You Some Kind of Witch Doctor?

FOR TWO YEARS after joining the running group, my gut beyond wrecked, I continued to run—with the moms, my friend Noel, and on my own. Bloated, cramping, doubled over on the curb, frantic for the next damn bathroom, I ran. And when I wasn't running, I was meeting with a boatload of medical practitioners and nutritionists who prescribed everything from L-Glutamine to iron to sublingual B-12. When it came to diet, I took the suggestions that made sense to me—no more gluten or dairy, and more pea-, rice- and hemp-based protein powders and bars to fill my animal protein void. Other suggestions, I completely dismissed. I refused to eat the amount of meat they suggested, or eggs for breakfast three times a week, or pasta (never a fan, much less the gluten-free variety), or the fruits and veggies I didn't like—plums, pears, tomatoes, potatoes, eggplant.

After about six months of nail biting and hopelessness, I finally got in to see a functional medicine practitioner whose waiting list was a mile long. I was elated. I'd heard great things. I just knew she was going to be the one with all the right answers. My time had finally come. I felt like I'd won the lottery! After a long initial consult, she ordered dozens of labs. When the results came back, we met again, and she sent me home with huge shopping bags filled with bottles of supplements, so many that I had to buy multiple pill boxes to organize them all, and write down the different times of day I needed to take each allocation. In retrospect, I should have made a freakin' spreadsheet. Juggling it all was like having another part-time job.

Since we agreed to follow an alternative path—no antibiotics—I believed these pills and supplements were going to be the answer to all my issues. Over the next several months, we continued to test and re-test, altering the supplement protocol based on the results of these labs. So many supplements. I cleared an entire shelf in my pantry to house the various bottles, tinctures, and powders. As I continued to swallow the pills, without seeing any change, Mark was watching the bills pile up, since the highly touted functional medicine doc I waited months to see did not take health insurance. Slowly, I began to accept that she was not my supplement superhero.

Sometimes these practitioners' prescriptions brought a bit of relief. Getting rid of gluten had been a good thing, and I think the protein powders and bars satiated me more than the rice cakes and almond butter/banana concoction I was constantly whipping together or, at least, they were a nice addition to my standard meal plan. I was also working with an amazing acupuncturist, Rosa, who recognized that my adrenals were off, my digestive fire was extremely low, and my yin-yang balance was far from equilibrium. When Rosa explained the theory of Chinese medicine and the properties of yin (the feminine,

inward flowing, right-brain energy) and yang (the masculine, outward flowing, left-brain energy), it was quite obvious I was *all* yang—
practical, logical, get-it-done. And I was extremely deficient in yin—
feelings, intuition, intimacy, imagination, at peace with what is. Yeah,
not me.

Rosa had a wonderful demeanor, and while she treated me, she'd
speak to me about my issues in a nonjudgmental, comforting manner. She offered several suggestions for foods, and occasionally recommended Chinese herbs and other supplements that I'd add to my
protocol. The treatments were something I looked forward to because
the time with her helped calm me down, allowing my body to rest
on her table for close to an hour. I tried to heed her advice regarding
my lifestyle. I asked her for suggestions about yoga. I confided in her.
She was a voice I could trust. She listened to all the diagnoses from
the various practitioners I saw through those years. And although
the acupuncture was helpful, the yoga was calming and restorative, the herbs, tinctures, and teas soothing, not one thing came
close to getting to the heart of my digestive problems, which were
making my life miserable.

It was unbelievably frustrating. I would do my best to keep my
cool on the outside, but on the inside I was losing it. I was losing hope
that someone could help me feel better. My frustration often turned
to anger, which I took out on those closest to me. The littlest things
would set me off. I had a no-tolerance policy when the kids left their
shoes on the floor, the sink was full of dishes, or I was stuck in traffic—these events would put me in an emotional tailspin. Most things I
could control, or change, or force to conform to my standards. But my
health issues were out of my hands, something I needed others to help

me navigate. I felt helpless, alone, and afraid that things were always going to be this way, or, G-d forbid, get worse! The constant physical reminders of bloat, distention in my belly, poop problems, and cramping just fed my anger, frustration, and depression.

Then somewhere along the line, after spending about two years in practitioners' waiting rooms, I read an article about Ayurvedic medicine. I believe that sometimes information presents itself to us at the most opportune times in our lives. Even if we don't initially realize why, there's a strong energetic force attracting us to it. Reading this article was certainly one of those times. I was immediately drawn to this holistic, ancient Indian medicine, with its focus on creating harmony among mind, body, and spirit. Ayurveda integrated herbal medicines, nutrition, meditation, exercise, and purification and rejuvenation therapies—holistically working to heal the body from within.

While reading the article, something clicked. I knew I needed to explore this science, this modality. It piqued my curiosity more than anything had in a very long time. I googled until I found a practitioner in Austin. I explored her website and read her bio. Kerry had studied for years with Vasant Lad, a famous Ayurvedic practitioner. Energetically, it felt like a good connection to make. My gut was telling me this Ayurveda thing was what I needed to explore for my healing. So with little more than a Google hit, a wish, and a prayer, I contacted Kerry for an appointment . . . ASAP.

The practitioners I'd been seeing had looked at my test results, but not at me. Kerry saw me. The appointment took place at my house, where she sat across from me at the kitchen table. Her energy was calming, her voice soothing, and her smile comforting. We chatted for about twenty minutes. I learned more about her history and her education, and she asked a few questions about my exercise routine, my sleep, my food (what I ate, and how frequently), my lifestyle, my habits. I described elements of myself—my temperament, personality traits, likes, dislikes. She asked to look at my hair, my nails, my skin, my tongue. She checked my pulse. And then she nailed me. *Completely*. Sure as shit. True AF. She got my personality, my body type, my behaviors, my sensitivities, and described them to a tee. She explained what was so out of whack about all these areas and what I needed to do to heal.

I was like, *Holy crap. She must be like some kind of wicked witch doctor, 'cause how else can she know all these things about me? And not just what's going on internally but about my whole personality. How could she know I'm stubborn? How could she know I'm impatient? How could she know I'm Type-A, driven? She read me like a book! You can't just look at a person and say that! I mean you could say, "Oh, I think you might have some digestive issues," or "You have really dry skin. Are you hydrating?"* She was able to describe, exactly, every single thing about the quality of my being and my personality. I was completely and totally blown away by her ability to do so. *WTF?!?!?!?* I was mentally kicking myself for not finding her sooner.

I must have looked stunned. "You're Vata-Pitta," she said.

I just stared at her. I had no idea what that meant. "Huh?"

She explained. In Ayurveda, there are three doshas, or mind-body energies. If the energies are out of balance, lethargy and depression can set in. You can be one single dosha and just express every element of that, or you can be a combination of two or even all three.

Vata is air. The driving force. It describes those who are in constant motion; they don't slow down, they thrive on chaos, adrenaline, and love to multi-task. They're runners. Their body types long and lean. They're cold-natured and usually dry. They're more inclined to eat lighter foods, cooler foods, raw foods. Too much wind or air or cold or raw will throw them off. Vata rules communication, creativity, flexibility, and quickness of thought. But too much Vata creates cold, constipation, crankiness, confusion. What a cluster-fuck!

Pitta is fire. Innately strong, intense, irritable, impatient, head-strong, extremely driven. They'll go after what they want in life. Pitta rules joy, courage, willpower, anger, jealousy, mental perception, sharp intellect. Positive traits can be a joyful disposition, a sharp intellect, and tremendous courage and drive. But if the fire gets too hot, anger, rashes, and ego can result. Burn, baby, burn!

Kapha is earth. It grounds Vata and Pitta. Kapha rules love, patience, forgiveness, greed, attachment, and mental inertia. This energy is strong and steady. Kapha people excel at endurance sports. (Kapha is my spirit animal.)

Before Kerry left, she once again stressed the importance of yoga, breathwork, and grounding, and mentioned the healing benefits of herbs and spices: ashwaganda, triphala, astragalus, manjistha, carda-mom, cumin, and tumeric. As I closed the front door behind her, I was already looking forward to our next session. As I learned more about Ayurveda and the three doshas, once again, a lightbulb came on. It *all* made sense to me. The more I pushed in the direction of Vata or Pitta, the further out of balance I would become. I didn't need more fire. I didn't need more air. The more salads I ate, the more miles I ran, the more events I chaired, the deeper I dug myself into the ditch. The effing ditch of feeling physically and emotionally like shit. All. The. Time!

In high school, I'd realized that many of my personality charac-
teristics—headstrong, driven, focused, determined, hot-tempered—
I'd inherited from my father (and his father). Though I didn't have a
name for it then, these are all Pitta traits. I now realized the connection was more than genetics; the similarities among us could all be
explained through the definition of the Ayurvedic doshas.

I met with Kerry once a week for more than a year. Our meetings revealed so much about my mindset and my body's makeup.
With my Vata-Pitta dosha, I had a lot more air and fire than I did
earth. Movement was not going to balance me. Sitting and meditating would, but I found this to be completely impossible. At the time,
it was a joke. I couldn't sit still for two seconds, much less twenty
minutes. Kerry told me my belly was too tight, always contracted,
and I needed to soften it and cultivate a softer approach to most
of the things in my life. I needed to B-R-E-A-T-H-E. Focus on my
inhales and exhales. Be more present in the moment and not always
so concerned about the next item on the agenda.

During our meetings, we sometimes practiced breathing exercises. Kerry tried
to get me to breathe into my belly.
She would instruct me to place
one hand on my lower abdomen and fill my abdomen
with air, watching my hand
rise and fall with each inhale

and exhale. In my head, I'd pooch out my belly, making it big, trying to create space in a place that was so knotted and tangled and held so many emotions. There was no way I was going to make my belly soft. I couldn't. It felt so foreign to even try, and even the one or two times Kerry said I did it right felt uncomfortable. I was tight and hard. It was part of my vanity.

Softening my belly was an exploration of an entirely new territory I didn't have the emotional strength to explore. I had no idea then how very important it was that I investigate this further.

Not only did Kerry introduce me to the importance of belly breathing (which I finally came back to, and which took years for me to accomplish), she also had a lot to say about my diet. Everything I was doing to fuel my body was only providing more of what I didn't need, which continued to push me in the wrong direction. As a Pitta, I was full of fire. Lots of fire, especially in my belly. So I needed a grounding diet. She knew I loved lots of spice. I was always adding heat—pepper, cayenne, tabasco—to my food to increase the intensity of the flavor, for more kick. Ya know, being from New Orleans and living in Texas, it was kind of a given. But that created too much heat, and Kerry wanted to cool that down. Plus I was eating a mostly raw food diet—tons of salad, raw veggies every day, cold foods, and smoothies with lots of raw greens. I never took the time to heat anything up, leftovers included. These foods were fueling my Vata and pushing me further away from center, and the equilibrium my body needed to achieve. Raw foods can be especially hard on people with a Vata constitution (who often have weak digestion) because they're harder to break down. Kerry told me I needed to eat cooked, warm, rooted foods, not cold, raw foods. Add warming spices (but not spicy)—cardamom, cumin, coriander, cinnamon, clove. Replace the raw fruits I was consuming with stewed fruits.

I was willing to try a few things she recommended, like making *kitcheri* (basmati rice, dal, and warm spices) for breakfast, adding some of her spices, and cooking my apples down once in a while, but that was it. The rest just didn't make sense to me. It wasn't until years later that I had an incredible moment, when I thought, *Wait. This so makes sense!* All the puzzle pieces starting fitting together and I could see the larger picture come into focus. I realized that's how I'd heal my belly. If I had such a compromised digestive system, then why would I keep forcing it to break down raw foods? Why wouldn't I start with pre-digested food like soup and broth? But at the time, I was like *What?* I didn't want to eat those foods or prepare those foods when I thought raw foods were so much easier and healthier.

As much sense as Kerry's advice made to me, and as intrigued as I was by the Ayurvedic principles of living, eating, and breathing, I wasn't willing to go to the places that scared me—tapering my running schedule, removing the raw veggies, going to bed earlier, meditating in the mornings, slowing down—it was all terrifying. Fundamentally, I didn't want to be soft. I literally couldn't stomach being open and vulnerable. That was something I was avoiding (sometimes consciously, sometimes unconsciously) at all costs. Pushing hard, keeping busy, running fast— it all provided the escape and distraction from dealing with the deep emotional and physical needs my body, in its rebellion over all these years, had been telling me I needed to recognize and honor.

Ayurveda resonated because it really, truly made sense on a foundational level. Something deep inside told me that this was the infrastructure I needed to build upon to improve my health, but my brain and gut weren't allowing me to assimilate it all because there was no connection there. The physical manifestations of my symptoms were my body yelling for change—to slow down, to stop running, to eat warm, pre-digested soups—but my brain kept firing messages to power through it all. I felt strong, invincible even. But I was far from invincible. My gut was way out of balance, which caused imbalances in my brain functions, hindering my cognitive abilities—I was far from focused, easily distracted, foggy brained. It took me a while to get things done, especially anything involving putting words together, whether I was writing a quick note to the kids, an email, a to-do list, or even speaking. I always felt the right word was on the tip of my tongue but my brain couldn't retrieve it. I had a hard time getting simple chores done. When I was grocery shopping or picking up a few things at Target, I'd forget why I was there or drift up and down the aisles in slow motion, wasting time because I had no strength. I felt exhausted. All the time. Yet, my fears were on overdrive. My thoughts raced; I was driven by self-doubt, fear, and uncertainty of what would lie ahead—the unknown. My brain had the upper hand and these thoughts were much more powerful than the signals bubbling up from below. My mind was constantly racing, which forced my body to follow suit, to run from the anxiety. But they both needed to rest and recover.

My relationships with Kerry and the other practitioners who'd also alluded to my mindset being part of the problem were one-sided. I couldn't listen to them. Every time a practitioner put me in a position of self-awareness, I'd simply shut down. When I was in their presence, in theory, what they were telling me made great sense, and I'd kind of tell myself I was going to make the change, or at least attempt to. But when I returned to my own environment, faced with my day-to-day habits, routines, and cravings, I'd ignore what they'd told me just days or hours before. I was too afraid to step out of my comfort zone and explore uncharted emotions, fearful of the physical transformations and conversations—both internal and with others—I'd have to confront. So, instead, I clung tightly to my habitual patterns, which prevented me from becoming a healthier version of myself. I kept paying them, going to appointments, and listening to their words and advice.

But it was just part of the whirlwind of reality that exemplified my health, which was more out of control than it had ever been. I'd been running away from these feelings for so long it was the only thing I knew how to do. I was a cyclist, swimmer, runner, personal trainer, group exercise instructor, fundraiser, house remodeler, triathlete, mom, wife, board member, room mom—the list went on as to how I defined myself and how others defined me. But then questions kept popping up in my mind: *How could I maintain all these personas and uphold the level I wanted to uphold? How could I be better than just good? Do we all hold ourselves accountable for more than we should? Do we need to excel in all areas?*

I strived for perfection in every single category. That's what I'd always done. That was my mantra. If I were to incorporate these practitioners' suggestions, my expectations of myself and those I perceived others were placing upon me were going to have to decrease.

What happens when we place too much pressure on ourselves? This self-induced pressure translates to stress. Stress is one of the biggest contributors to our mental and physical well-being. We can eat right and exercise all we want, but if we continue to live under a bubble of stress day in and day out, we'll eventually create our own demise. We teach our children to learn from their mistakes. Why don't we grant ourselves that same allowance? We learn and grow from each and every failure in life, becoming stronger and developing thicker skin. So when we're down, why not just pick ourselves up off our asses and start all over again? Brush it off, baby. No one else gives a flying fuck that we failed! But instead, we often beat ourselves up, become depressed, compare ourselves to others we believe excel more easily in certain roles—because they do more, know more, and do it better. My drive and my ambition were tangled up in the perceptions I thought others were placing on me. That shit was all made up. Those self-induced projections drove me crazy, kept me striving to be the best at my game. I thought that was what everyone else expected, so if I didn't meet those expectations, I'd fail.

For years, I continued to run with my poor gut screaming at me to stop. But I always had to finish. And finish strong. Because what if I didn't? I would #fail. That's what we're all fearful of, right? We don't want to fail. We have been taught by society not to. It's kind of taboo, yeah? Well, let me tell you. Failure has been my best friend. Recognizing that perfection is not achievable, that the perfect volunteer or mom or athlete status doesn't exist. Meeting my unrealistic expectations and beating myself up for not achieving them was how I associated my actions with failure. Yet looking back, those failures were my greatest strength. They taught me to move forward and embrace my best effort, no matter what the outcome. Stop making excuses. When you can admit you were wrong, when you take two (or ten) steps backward to move forward, and when you begin to recognize that perfection is not reality, then and only then will you begin to heal.

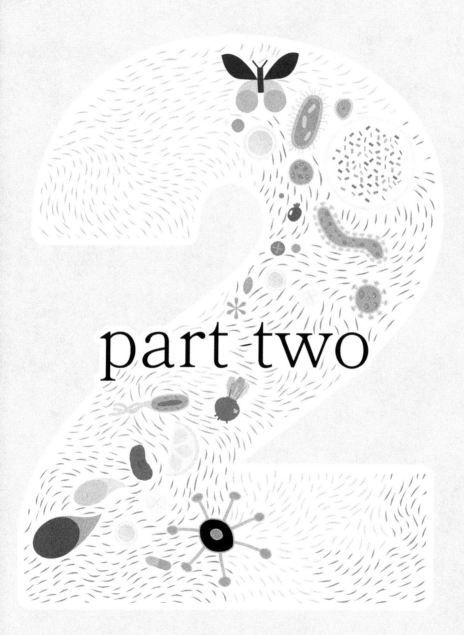

part two

When Working Out Stopped Working Out

How are you feeling?

Another marathon?!

You're TOO thin...

THROUGHOUT 2009, I continued to consult with nutritionists and practitioners about my gut, which was still a wreck even after numerous attempts to repair the damage. They would take one look at me and resort to packing in calories and adding even more supplements, which didn't work, because most of what they suggested were a bunch of foods and pills that my body wasn't absorbing anyway. How could it? Nothing stayed in my system long enough. These people weren't listening to me, which really pissed me off because, by that point, I'd done research, I had some idea of what I was talking about. Still, I understood why they blew me off. First, I looked like shit. Hair, skin, nails—all dry. Complexion gray. Lanky, muscular, but far too thin. I needed to gain weight, yesterday. And second, I knew that as soon as they saw me, they thought: anorexia.

I fit the picture of the stereotypical fitness fanatic who is dealing with exercise addiction and eating issues, someone whose thinking is fairly warped. But I was far from anorexic. I wasn't afraid of eating. I ate plenty. The main fear surrounding my eating habits stemmed from my belly's reaction to the foods I ate—pretty much any food. Sometimes it was several minutes, other times hours, before the gas and bloating set in. At these times, as anyone can imagine, it was uncomfortable being around people. The flatulence started like a fuckin' symphony and my bowels could erupt at any freakin' minute. Vanity did enter into it for sure, but mainly if what I ate made me feel awful—big, heavy, and so bloated that I couldn't exercise as often or as hard—then I wouldn't want to eat as much. So I ate very little before my workouts. I had very little fuel to burn when I chose to exert myself, and then, upon completing some of those intense sessions, my ravenous body would actually start to cannibalize my muscle as fuel, placing me in a larger deficit. Any attempt to refuel and repair wasn't happening. The food and the exercise got tangled up in this mental and physical web that kept my body in a constant state of depletion. And it certainly looked it.

My parents worried. I would frequently hear: "How are you feeling?" "You're too thin." "Why do you need to run another marathon?" Several times, my mom mentioned that her friends had made comments to her. They told her I looked sickly and too thin. They, too, wondered what was going on and whether I needed help. My mom's friends weren't the only ones who were chiming in. My friends also made comments. But most of them chose to speak to Mark, not directly to me.

Concerned, Mark started to watch me more closely—what I ate and when, how much I exercised. He even walked in on me one time doing jumping jacks in the bathroom. I often caught a few minutes here and there throughout the day because I felt I needed to get in just a bit more exercise, every day just a bit more. It also helped with my anxiety, allowing me to pound out my fears and frustrations. And it released pent-up emotions I couldn't express. I felt mortified when he caught me. *Soooo* embarrassed! It was stupid (seriously, why was I jumping around in the bathroom?) if I thought about it, which I did, for a minute, but that didn't stop me the next time.

Mark could see how thin I was. At the same time, he knew I wasn't starving myself. I wasn't sitting at dinner, staring at the single pea on my plate, trying to get it to last an hour. I ate a lot. Just the wrong foods. I was constantly hungry because everything I ate was basically carbohydrates with a small amount of protein thrown in for good measure. I ate quinoa, popcorn, a lot of raw veggies, and the staple of my diet was rice cakes. The carbs seemed to help absorb all of the gurgling and gook that was swimming around in my stomach. I kept my homemade trail mix in my purse or the glove compartment of my car. I constantly nibbled because I always felt hungry. Always! I kept sleeves of rice cakes in my car and a hefty supply at home to alleviate my irrational fear that Lundberg's factory would shut down and I wouldn't be able to find them anywhere. When I wasn't munching on rice cakes in my car, I sat at my kitchen island, slathering them with nut butter and topping them with sliced bananas. Sleeves at a time until my hunger finally began to subside. There obviously wasn't enough animal protein in my diet. On some level I knew that, but I couldn't make myself eat animal protein, except for seafood every now and then. It was a mental thing as well as a physical thing. My digestive system didn't have the strength or

capacity to handle large amounts of animal protein at the time—it
had been a foreign substance for so long.

I kept on like this. Then one day, I got home from a run, and
in all my sweatiness, went to the kitchen to get something to eat.
Mark followed me in. "What are you doing tomorrow?" he asked. I
shrugged, my head in the fridge. "I don't know. I'll probably go run
with Noel in the morning." He asked if I had plans after that. I told
him I didn't, then asked him why he wanted to know. "Because your
parents want to come over," he said, "and they want to talk to you,
with me."

Wait. "What? Why with the three of you?"

"They want to discuss some things with you with me there."

I was starting to feel angry and became totally defensive. "What
the eff is going on?"

"You tell me," he said. "Your mom's been calling me at work. She's
concerned that you're too thin, that you exercise too much. They want
to come over to talk with you. She said you need to be spoken with
and she wanted us all together, but they're going to talk to you with or
without me."

I freaked out. What was I, ten? In the state I was in, I felt my parents were intruding on my life, my marriage. I slammed the door to
the fridge and threw my water bottle across the room toward the sink,
as if I *were* ten. I was so pissed off. I couldn't believe my parents had
set this up behind my back.

"What about the kids?" I asked. "I don't want them here." But I
didn't need to worry. Turned out my sister, Karen, was taking them,
which infuriated me even more. They'd pulled her in too?

"She has no idea what's going on," Mark said quickly.

That was bullshit, and I knew it. Mark might believe that, but I knew better—my sister had a one-year-old, and there's no way my mom would ask her to take our kids without telling her why she needed her help.

I was yelling, swearing, crying. I felt not only betrayed but afraid, anxiety swirling within me. Sure, I was hurt, but I felt completely helpless. I couldn't control the situation, I couldn't control my health issues, and no professional I had consulted was able to either. I was out of excuses and my back was up against a wall. A big, brick wall and there was no getting past it, no matter how headstrong I was. Things were starting to unravel before my eyes. I felt alone and unsupported, though that's exactly the antithesis of what was happening—I just didn't realize it at the time.

The hunger pangs I'd felt when I'd returned from my workout completely vanished. I felt nauseated, a tight wad of nerves in my belly. Mark kept his distance. He looked stern and wasn't going to take any of my business this time. At that point, he'd started putting all the pieces together and knew something was wrong. And while he didn't yet realize the complexity or the level to which things had escalated, his concerns rose as my weight declined and my issues became more complex —emotionally, mentally, and physically.

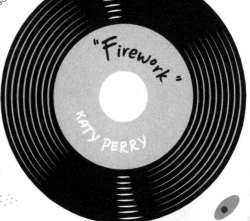

"I don't get any of this," I said. "What are they going to do? Ground me?"

Mark told me to call them and talk to them, but I didn't. I felt exhausted and emotionally drained. I resigned myself to the fact that this was going to happen—no ifs, ands, or buts. I was just like, "Whatever happens, happens. They can come over."

Mark called them and they decided to come over later that day. So I showered, and then waited, my poor sad belly in knots, dreading what I knew would be a difficult and painful meeting.

We met in the kitchen, the air thick with tension. I felt my body stiffen. I was already starting to put up my line of defense. Because that's how I roll, or used to. I sat at one end of our long kitchen table. My parents sat on one side and Mark sat across from them. My mom had pages of notes in front of her. My dad had his yellow legal pad (he loves yellow legal pads) filled with his notes. They started very softly.

"Ellen," my dad said, "we love you very much. We're so proud of you, but we're very concerned that you aren't healthy. You don't look well; you're exercising too much, in our opinion."

My mom looked up from her notes. "We think there's something the matter. You look very thin, and our friends see you and comment on it, and your friends, too. There's a lot of conversation about what's going on with Ellen."

A lot of conversation? That shocked me. I knew people had been making comments, but not to that extent. I sat very still. Humiliated, furious, defensive. I felt this was not the way they ought to be to handling their concerns. I bit my lip. Then things got worse. Mark had been sitting there quietly all along. He's quiet to begin with, especially around confrontation, especially confrontation between my parents and me. I'm sure he was scared shitless. I can't remember how much he said during the meeting. I do remember him saying, "Ellen, don't yell. We've all talked about this. You've been exercising a lot, not eating enough, and we've all been concerned." But not much else. My parents pretty much ran the show.

I took a deep breath. "If you wanted to talk to me about this, you could have definitely chosen a different platform."

"Ellen, we've tried. Many times, we've tried," my mom said, "and you don't listen. We're demanding that you get help."

Demanding?

"We're insisting—"

Insisting? Are you freakin' kidding me?

"You go see an eating disorders specialist."

My mom handed me a piece of paper with some names jotted down. "Susan gave me names here in Austin that she would recommend for you." Susan, my mom's good friend from high school, was a nutritionist who specialized in eating disorders (my mom had consulted her when I was in high school running cross-country). Bringing Susan in felt like déjà vu, but this time I was married with kids and adult enough to make my own decisions. Well, not necessarily, as it turned out.

There was a lot of drama, that's for sure. They were in *my* house telling *me* what I *had* to do. The discussions surrounding my health went far beyond that kitchen table—my sister, my friends, my mom's friends, who else? I was curious. I began to feel like this whole group of people was ganging up against me and I had to fight to defend myself—alone. I started freaking out. I couldn't believe it. I couldn't hold on to my emotions anymore.

I yelled and screamed at them. I swore. A lot. At some point, I stopped, waited a second, trying to calm down and catch my breath, shocked at the words that had just come out of my mouth.

"I hear that you care for me. I hear that you love me, that you're doing this out of concern for me, for my well-being and my health, but I resent how it's being done. I think your delivery is extremely poor, and if you're 'demanding' and 'insisting' that I see someone then I will go about it on my own terms. I will go and find the practitioner myself without your help." I shoved the piece of paper back toward my mother. "I'll only go see someone I feel comfortable seeing. Period."

At that point, there wasn't much more to discuss. We were all worn out, completely spent. I cried like a baby and knew deep down that this was all coming from a place of love and caring for their daughter and wife who was sliding down a slippery slope. I knew I needed help, but hearing it from them, in that manner, brought up so much fear, so much pain, such a feeling of helplessness. I didn't want to show my vulnerabilities, my weaknesses, and I damn sure wasn't going to give in. My control issues were overriding all the emotions that were surfacing. I wouldn't give in. Once again I did what I had taught myself to do so well: I dug deep to push through the pain. But this time it was emotional, not physical pain. We ended the meeting with hugs but very few words. I didn't storm out, though I had very little left to say. I had so many feelings—but expressing myself in words was just not happening.

My parents and husband love me very much. I know that, and I love them with all my heart. They'd never, ever do anything to intentionally hurt or harm me, or anyone else. I don't blame anyone for what happened. This was truly an expression of love and concern for my health. It needed to happen, I just didn't realize it at the time. I was forced to step into a reality that I wasn't ready to face head on and it hurt like hell.

My feelings during that discussion formed a tornado of swirling emotions and, at some point, it felt like a lightning bolt pierced right through me, shaking me up and sending an electric current to my brain. My head was clouded with fear, rage, and denial. And the denial that I needed help, that I needed to stop, that I needed to slow down was real to me. Now more than ever before. And it was so effing scary. I was absolutely *not* ready to hear what they had to say. Deep down inside, I knew it was coming. I knew it was something I needed to hear. I knew I needed to be forced into a corner in order to take action. Because, I *am* a force to be reckoned with sometimes! My head can get too jaded, strong, and egotistical. I like to be in control of my own destiny and navigate my own course. I don't like others telling me what to do and when to do it, even when I know they're right. I needed to get over that, and fast.

Hips Don't Lie

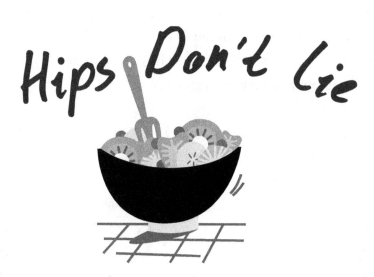

AS IF ONE intervention wasn't enough—boom!—about three months later, I was hit with another one. This time it was my running group that stepped up, but this one felt much different. I didn't feel blindsided—maybe because the relationship I had with these women had been all about support, ever since the day I met them, while the relationship with my family is tangled up with love, fear, and years of history. These girls were runners, moms, intensity junkies, and we had a mutual love of exercise. The honesty, integrity, and authenticity of these women amazes me to this day.

One day as I was driving, I got a call from Paige, one of the women in the group.

"I need to talk to you," Paige said. "We need to talk to you. By "we," she meant her, her BFF Kristin, and Cassie, our running coach. "Something's the matter," she said. "You don't look well. You're way too thin, and we're concerned about you."

I didn't say a word. I wasn't angry, but my heart was pounding. It felt as though I'd been caught eating a protein bar in the aisle of Whole Foods and ditching the evidence in my purse. I felt I'd been found out as a fraud by a group of very authentic women I so admired.

"We want to go out to lunch, and we want you to tell us what's going on with you. We want to help."

Lunch? My stomach dropped.

Before I could say anything, Paige told me about a friend of hers, Janet, whom she wanted me to meet—a marathon runner who'd struggled with and overcome anorexia. She'd continually lost weight, until she was really, really thin. Her doctor advised her many times to stop running, but she continued to run, getting thinner and thinner, until one day she almost died running a marathon.

"She knows the signs," Paige said. "And if she sees those same signs with you, she'll be able to talk with you about it."

I listened attentively. Convincing people that I wasn't anorexic when I looked so gaunt and frail was a challenge. It appeared that they had collectively made up their minds that I was dealing with this condition and they wanted to help. The complexity of my situation was difficult to explain. I could still race. I wasn't collapsing. I could still run fast, push myself harder, and was PR'ing (personal record) my races, achieving my best times. But it was true. I was thin, too thin.

My messed-up body image would change by the day or by the hour. Some days, I'd get out of the shower, and think, *Oh, my G-d. You're so freaking thin. Too freaking thin. Put some meat on your bones, girl! That's not appealing. Curves are sexy!* And then, poof! As the thought of sexy curves triggered fear and anxiety for me, the desire to gain weight would evaporate like the condensation on the mirror left from my shower. I'd move the internal discussion to *I'm not too thin . . . yet.* Then I'd look in the mirror, get dressed, and it was almost like nothing had entered my mind. I actually thought I looked fine: *Nothin' to worry about. Nope, I'm all good!*

Paige continued talking about her friend. So far, I hadn't said a word. Paige wasn't giving me a chance, which was fine with me. I had no idea how to respond.

"She was admitted to a rehab facility for a few months after nearly dying during the race," Paige said. "She's still working at it, but she's in a good place now. I really want you to meet with her. But first, I want the four of us to meet for lunch: Kristin, Cassie, you, and me."

I felt touched that they were concerned, that they wanted to help. As afraid as I was, I was just as humbled by the fact that these women cared enough about me to put themselves in this uncomfortable position. Plus, deep down, I knew something was wrong. They could see through me, read between the lines of my convoluted stories, warped self-concept, and rationalizations. They could see what I couldn't. I trusted them. So I agreed to meet them at 24 Diner, a restaurant that offered local, sustainable, inspired comfort food.

When I got to the diner, they were already seated. They waved. I walked to the table, a total wreck. And right away, they didn't mess around, they just hit me with it. "Hey, Ellen. We're concerned about you and your health. You're really thin. We've seen you whittle down in size over the last several months. We've been running together for a while now and it's obvious that something's the matter. We want you to continue running with us. We really like you. You're a great person, and we've loved getting to know you. We really want to talk to you about whatever it is that's going on. We're here to support you and help you through whatever you need." Paige and Kristin were doing most of the talking, attempting to create a comfortable space in which I could share, assuring me that whatever I said was in confidence, and that their concern and friendship were the reason for our meeting. Cassie was watching and listening attentively, chiming in here and there, though of the three, she was the quietest.

My relationship with Cassie felt different than the relationship I had with Kristin and Paige. Cassie was the coach. She wasn't in the trenches running with us. I suppose those workouts created a deeper bond between Page, Kristin, and me. We ran together, struggled through the intervals together, and cheered each other on. We shared the pain and the triumph. I could relate to them more and they to me. Still, Paige and Kristin were much closer with Cassie than I was. The three of them were friends outside the run group. I expect Cassie was there to provide a different perspective (that of a coach), while the other two seemed concerned on an emotional level.

I leaned forward, hands folded on the table. I felt so nervous and on edge. I was very reserved and quiet compared to the usual exuberance I generally displayed around them. I knew they were right. That little voice in my head was shrieking: *Something's wrong. You better listen. You're too thin. You need to stop doing the jumping jacks in the bathroom. You need to stop running when your body's telling you not to. You need to change your diet and listen to your body telling you you're not getting enough. Why else do you think you're never satiated?* I wanted and needed to open up, to let them help me, to admit something deeper was going on, beyond just the issues with my gut. But I just couldn't. I felt too afraid.

"I have a lot of stomach issues," I said.

There was an uncomfortable silence. They all nodded. I knew they had more to say, but they didn't go into it right then. Instead we picked up our menus. I felt a feeling of "all eyes on me." They were watching to see what I'd order, trying not to be too obvious, probably thinking, *What's it going to be? Will she finish it? C'mon, Ellen, prove to me that you don't have an eating disorder!*

I ordered fruit salad. How's that for weak, scared, and confirming the obvious? I don't remember what they ate, but more than a freakin' fruit salad for sure. I was so nervous about what was about to go down that any and all hunger pangs had been totally quashed. "There are certain things I can't eat," I said. "Certain foods upset my stomach terribly. And so I've really been forced to hone in on which foods work and which don't. I can't eat dairy or gluten or red meat. All those things upset my belly." They already knew I had issues with these foods. That wasn't what they wanted to hear. There was no one I could convince that my issues weren't limited to an eating disorder— they, like my parents, were convinced I must be anorexic.

Paige spoke about how strong and muscular I looked when I had first joined the running group. She thought I was the epitome of a triathlete—long, lean, and always looking to improve. Kristin told me how impressed she was with my accomplishments. She'd seen a marked improvement in my times since I'd started with the group. She and I were always about the same pace, and instead of competition, it felt more like comradery, even when we were panting in each other's ears while circling the track together. They were alarmed by the steady decline in my size from the time they'd met me, not quite two years earlier. Cassie, although reserved in her comments, chimed in and said she thought I no longer looked healthy. She could see the veins popping out on my arms and legs when I ran. She eluded to the fact that the food restrictions, coupled with the intense exercise, were not a good combination. She strongly advised me to seek help. Paige and Kristin agreed. They all spoke directly from the heart, at times very gently, at others more sternly, but I always heard their concern and support. Cassie, too, was somewhat gentle, though less so than the others. That's just how she is—tough, tense. She doesn't take BS from anyone. Not even the homeless men at the park who would catcall to us when we were running intervals. Once, she pranced her petite little self over to where they sat at a picnic table and told them to stop yelling and leave. And they did! I was in awe.

Mostly, I sat and listened, and thought, *Wait a minute. They're really smart. They've nailed me, right? They got me.* I felt trapped between a rock and a hard place; they were confronting me with real issues, but there was also something much deeper going on. And though I listened to them, believed them, respected them, I kept getting caught up in all the other bullshit that was going through my head. I wanted to admit to them that they were right, that there was something deeper going on that had to do with appearance, performance, control. I wanted to tell them how important they were to me and how their authenticity, grace, and friendship had made such an impression, such a difference in my life. These women were exactly who I strived to be: strong, both mentally and physically, genuine, selfless. No phoniness here. But instead of emulating them and admitting I needed help, I froze up inside. Fear, pride, and embarrassment overcame truth and my response was one big hashtag: #FAIL. I couldn't fess up. I was too afraid. I knew they could read between the lines and I felt that I was quickly losing their respect. I was one big burrito of bullshit.

I left the meeting feeling a little dazed and confused. Not about the conversation, but about my own feelings. I was anxious that things would no longer be the same between us. They were onto something. They shot straight from the hip and expected me to do the same. I was being held accountable on a different level, and I cared too much about these women to let them down.

I agreed to meet Paige's friend Janet. That was my olive branch. I called her and we met at a coffee shop a few weeks later. I recognized her right away, although we'd never met. She looked like a waif, just tiny. I looked at her and thought she was too thin. Surprisingly, it didn't even cross my mind that people looked at me and thought the same thing. She told me her story, how she'd almost died running a marathon that her doctor had instructed her not to do. After that incident, her husband and kids insisted she go to a clinic for eating disorders. Now, she said, she was in a place where she could sit down and eat dinner with her family. In fact, her kids would call her out if she didn't. They'd also call

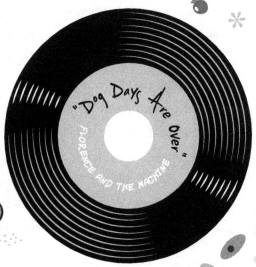

her out if she did anything that resembled old "ED" (eating disorder) behavior. "Mom," they'd say, "ED is here."

I recognized much of what she described in myself. I wasn't eating with my family. It felt like, at least when I did, that I was living out an old Police song: "Every move you make, every breath you take, I'll be watching you." It was hard for me to have a conversation at a meal because I constantly felt eyes staring at my plate. I was so self-conscious of each and every bite I took. It was an emotional see-saw of wanting the connection with my family but feeling too awkward and unnerved to sit down with them. I was very conscious of my behavior. Eating had become such an uncomfortable space for me. It made me feel insecure in my body. The bloat would come on almost immediately, then the gas, then the rumblings down below. I didn't want to be around anyone when that happened. It wasn't pretty and it certainly didn't make me feel pretty. I felt gross, large, on edge—those feelings inside my gut triggered depressing thoughts in my head. My frustrations would begin to surface, my mind would race with negative thoughts about myself, and I basically turned into a bitch. So, instead of being around my family when that happened, I chose to eat separately and just deal with it on a one-on-one basis—me and my gut at war once again. Not eating with my family made me feel isolated, confused, and alone, but my brain couldn't decipher the difference between what I should and shouldn't do. I knew deep down that sitting and sharing a meal was more important, but the fear and anxiety of doing so prevailed. The guilt would set in, and then it would happen all over again.

At the end of my conversation with Janet, she gave me the name of her therapist and suggested that I go see her. I left feeling a bit apprehensive, though my accountability circle—running group, family, practitioners, all of whom expected me to listen and carry through on my word to follow advice—kept expanding, so I followed through the way I always do when I say I'm going to do something. I didn't want to let anyone down, nor would I go back on my word. I knew deep inside that my issue wasn't the same as Janet's. While I definitely had food issues—orthorexia, wanting to eat only good, clean, healthy food—the origin was entirely different from anorexia. My eating disorder stemmed from my gut issues, which messed with my head, until I was caught in a vicious loop. Our headspace was similar, though—we both had eating disorders, and I was hopeful that the woman she referred me to would be able to help. I went home and set up an appointment, and then called Janet to thank her for meeting with me. I told her I had scheduled a meeting with her therapist and thanked her again for giving me the name, and for her concern.

My memories of the meetings with this therapist are foggy. I do know that on my first appointment, I was far from blown away. I spent the entire hour talking to her about my condition, my gut issues, and my food restrictions, so forming an opinion wouldn't be playing fair. When I came home Mark asked me how things went. "I didn't get that love connection," I said, but I agreed to go back again. Maybe I would warm up to her on a consecutive visit, right? Yeah, well, that didn't happen. Nope, not even close. After another two or four or however many more meetings, I determined that she and I were not exactly a Bumble match.

Honestly, I did try to make it work. I wanted it to work, especially since Janet had recommended her and they'd had so much success working together. Plus, I'd told Paige I was seeing her.

My intervention from the running moms caused me to listen more deeply to that little whisper that was coming from within. What they shared—their gentle approach and their desire to help me, an outsider, a newbie, a soul sister in need—really showed their integrity, their authenticity, and their love. They cared, and that meant a lot to me. Especially in a moment when everything else was coming undone.

Me, Myself, and My Gut

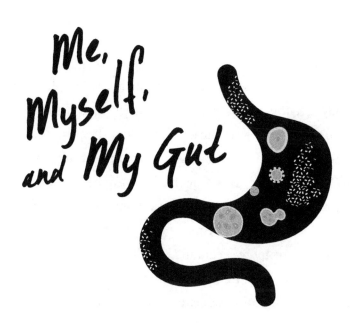

IT'S THE THINGS that happen randomly, that come at you from left field, that often stop life in its tracks. Everything changes in an instant, and you realize you're no longer in control. Because, truly, you never really were (even if your badass self had other ideas). Everything. Everything can unravel in an instant. March 12, 2010, was one of the times.

It was the Thursday before my kids' spring break, and I'd felt bad all day. During my daughter's gymnastics performance, I'd laughed and chatted with my friends, but I kept thinking, *Oh my G-d, my stomach really hurts.* It was bloated far more than it normally was. I brought the kids home from school, made dinner, and after dinner, I sent them to get ready for bed. The pain hadn't subsided, but I didn't let on to Mark or the kids. I'm not one to show pain. I did the dishes hunched over the sink because my stomach hurt so much. This pain was more intense than what I'd been feeling for the past three years—much more than gas pain. It was deep. Deep stomach pain.

Somehow, I finished cleaning up, made the kids' lunches for the next day, got them into bed, then dragged myself to bed at about eleven o'clock. Mark was already asleep, but the pain was so intense, I couldn't drift off. I kept tossing and turning, tossing and turning—on my belly, on my side, on my back, to my belly again. I got up to go to the bathroom. That didn't work. I still felt that stuck and gassy feeling inside, but nothing would release. I got back in bed, and tossed and turned some more. I couldn't lie still. I got up out of bed, walked around the bedroom, then went into the den and sat on the couch. Sitting didn't relieve the pain either. I crawled onto the floor and bent into a modified child's pose, my poor distended stomach hard as a rock. I lifted my butt in the air and thought for sure that this position would let one fly and release some pressure. It had worked for me before, but not this time. I felt as though someone had inflated a balloon inside my belly. I got back in bed. Midnight, 1:00, 1:30. I alternated between bathroom and bed, bathroom and bed. I was angry with my body. I needed sleep. The pain was searing. I didn't know what to do, but I didn't want to wake up Mark. I kept thinking, *He's a lawyer, not a doctor.* And he needs his sleep.

But finally, in tears, I got up, walked around to his side of the bed, tapped him on the shoulder, and woke him up.

He opened his eyes. "What is it?"

"My stomach really hurts. I have these horrible pains in my side and abdomen. I don't know what's wrong." I dropped to my knees, crawled over to the rug at the foot of our bed and curled up in a fetal position.

He sat up, threw off the covers. "I'm calling 911."

"You're *not* calling 911," I yelled from the floor. I was in my mental marathon mode. I could push through this. I'd never experienced this level of pain, not even in childbirth, but calling 911 seemed like such a loser thing to do. Instead, I lay there in agony. I wanted to battle this pain and take it head on. I wanted to beat this motherfucker up! Just like everything else, I thought I was bigger than the pain. I could overcome it. I would prevail. I refused to believe that I could not overcome this pain the way I'd overcome the pain during countless races.

Finally, I decided to call my OB/GYN. I asked Mark to hand me the phone. I dialed the doctor's office and was forwarded to the on-call service. After giving them my name and a few details about the situation, they told me the doctor on call would get back with me shortly. A few minutes later she called back and told me that my symptoms didn't sound like an obstetrics or gynecological issue at all. She told me to call 911. I hung up, thinking, *Oh, my G-d. I'm so dumb.* Then I started dry heaving from the pain.

Mark freaked out. "That does it. I'm calling 911!"

"You're not calling 911," I yelled between dry heaves. "I'm not talking to them." I would have stood up, but I couldn't pull my knees from my chest at that point.

Mark grabbed a pair of jeans. "Then I'm taking you to the ER!"

By that point, I was in so much pain that I didn't argue. It didn't stop me from getting really angry though. "I can't move. And you can't pick me up in this fetal position. There's no way."

"Then I'm calling 911."

I still clutched the phone. "*I'll* call them." I dialed 9-1-1.

While I was on the phone with the dispatcher, Mark called my mom on his cell and asked her to come stay with the kids.

The dispatcher asked for my location, then began a series of questions. "Tell me what's going on?"

I answered the questions, then said sternly, "Listen to me. I live on a cul-de-sac with two other houses. If you're sending somebody over here, I don't want any sirens. Do you understand?" Then I bent over and threw up.

"How long has your pain been going on?"

I wiped my mouth with the back of my hand. "All day, pretty much, but the pain keeps getting worse. It's intolerable. But did you get what I said? Don't turn on the lights. Don't turn on the sirens. Please!" I didn't want anybody to know what was going on and I didn't want to wake my kids.

This went on. She'd ask a question, I'd tell her no sirens. She'd ask another one, I'd tell her no flashing lights. Everything was a blur after that. I don't think it could have been ten minutes later when I looked up and saw Mark standing next to two men with a stretcher. They obviously wanted to get me from the floor to the stretcher, but I peeped my head up like a turtle from my ball-like position on the floor and explained, as nicely as I could, that there was *no fucking way* I could straighten my legs. One of the guys told me not to worry, then he pulled out a large syringe and gave me a shot in the hip.

"There," he said. "That will help to relax the muscles in your body so we can get you onto the stretcher." They both picked me up, one by the shoulders and one by my legs, placed me on my side on the stretcher, still balled up with my knees to my chest, then wheeled me through the house and into the ambulance. After that,

76

it was a bit of a blur again. I remember Mark poking his head into the ambulance, giving me a kiss and telling me he'd follow us over after my mom arrived. She was on her way. I do know the kids didn't wake up, and I thank G-d for that.

Once we arrived at the hospital, I was wheeled straight into an ER room and saw the first of what would be a long line of doctors. Once Mark arrived, he came into the room while they hooked me up to various machines, tubes, IVs, and monitors. I was coherent and lay relatively quietly while Mark spoke to the team of doctors and nurses about the chain of events that had brought us there. Then he filled out mounds of paperwork.

They began to ask me questions—what seemed like millions of them: "When did your pain start?" "Does it hurt here?" "How about here?" "When's the last time you had anything to eat or drink?" "What's your pain level on a scale of one to ten?" And in between questions, a nurse checked my vitals. "We're going to do some testing, have one of our ER docs come in and take a look at you, and make a determination about how we're going to move forward."

I was asked if I wanted morphine for my pain. *Morphine? Isn't that a high-level narcotic that's crazy addictive? I don't do drugs. I don't need morphine. I don't even take antibiotics for an infection. That sounds too extreme. These docs don't know who they're dealing with.* I refused.

The doctor warned me that there would be a series of tests run to figure out where the distension, pain, and nausea were stemming from. Some of these tests were going to be uncomfortable. I think one of my IVs was administering pain meds, though my pain was so severe that I couldn't think or focus on anything else. I felt nauseated, as though I was going to puke again, so after my initial refusal of the morphine, I didn't have the wherewithal to protest any other meds. I needed something to take the edge off. Anything. *Bring it! And fast!*

The next thing I knew two nurses wheeled in this contraption—similar to an IV pole, but instead of the clear bag usually hanging from the hook, there was a bright yellow plastic device that looked like an old-school, waterproof Sony Walkman. It had a lock and key plus a keypad. And tubes hung from it—multiple tubes—that the nurses were trying to stick into my arm.

I looked at them. "What is that thing?"

One of them rattled off some name that sounded like a word I had learned in seventh grade Latin class. "I don't know what that means," I said.

"It's an extremely powerful painkiller."

"Yeah, well why does it have its own prison cell?"

They said it was ten times more potent than morphine. It's the most stolen drug in hospitals, and the most highly addictive. Holy shit! But by that point, I was all in. The stronger the better. Bring it! I found out later that two people had to administer this drug for accountability. One of them had the key. The other had the keycode. After a few minutes, one of them asked me how I was feeling, and to my surprise, I was a bit more relaxed. It had taken the edge off, though I still felt a deep pain in my abdomen. I had managed to pull my legs away from my belly just a bit, though I was still in a somewhat twerked fetal position.

Another nurse came at me with a clear plastic cup (and we're not talking Dixie cup) full of some red sugary substance, held it to my mouth, and told me to drink it. It smelled like Kool-Aid. I looked at her. *What the fuck?!?* I told her I couldn't even think of drinking anything, not even water. I was too nauseated. "I'll barf," I said. But they insisted. I pointed at Mark to bring me a trashcan. He went to reach for it under the bedside table and tried to get it to me, but as soon as I took a sip, I puked all over myself.

The nurses cleaned me up, and although I was still curled up in a sideways dead bug position, they tried to get me into a hospital gown. I was quite little at the time—thin and frail—so my belly looked awkward and disproportionate to the rest of my body, like I was five months pregnant. Although the drugs were making me woozier by the minute, the expressions on their faces and the looks they gave each other as they gingerly placed my torso into the gown alarmed me.

They got a drip going after several stabs at my veins trying to find one that worked, then started in on the bloodwork. It seemed they were always drawing blood. Poking at my uncooperative veins that refused to give up the fight. *OMG, puh-leeze!* I thought. *I'm in enough pain. Let's do this, people!* But they said my veins were rolling and every time they went to take a stab at them, they moved. I was pissed off but kept trying to keep my shit together, ya know, as I do so very well! So I just chose to grit my teeth, smile, and let my emotions roll right along with my veins.

Next, a tech came in to wheel me out of the room for a CT scan. He was really friendly, talking the whole time, outlining the process. *Fine. Whatever.* I was ready to get on with this. Then I saw the machine—a big white igloo-looking machine they were going to bring over my mid-section.

Seriously, how was my curled up, contorted body getting into that thing? "I need you to straighten out your knees," the tech said.

"I can't."

"I'm going to need you to straighten your knees, so we can get you into the machine."

"I can't straighten my knees. I can't straighten my knees." *Which part of I CAN'T STRAIGHTEN MY KNEES do you not understand?!?!?*

He tried to straighten them for me. He manipulated my feet away from my butt and started extending my legs. I thought I was going to die. I really thought I was going to die. I was in so much excruciating pain. It totally felt as though my insides were going to tear apart. Thinking back, if he'd pulled on my legs too hard and my insides did tear, I could have died. Fo shizzle.

Finally, he got me into the thing. "Don't breathe," he said. "Don't move."

Believe me, I didn't breathe. I didn't move. My belly hadn't ripped, which was good, but I'm surprised I didn't pass out from holding my breath. All I could think was, *When is this going to be over?* The machine rotated around my midsection. With every fiber of my being, I wanted to pull my knees to my chest, but I had to keep them extended. I struggled to stay strong, focused, and determined that I would get through this. *Don't cave. Don't move. Don't breathe. You can do this!* I tapped into that same strength and tenacity I was so accustomed to channeling during my races, but this time, it was a matter of life or death.

After reviewing my X-rays, the radiologist and the first ER doctor I saw thought there was an obstruction in my colon, so they ordered a colonoscopy to remove it. Their thinking was that the colonoscopy would relieve the obstruction and, therefore, my pain. I'd had my first and only colonoscopy a few years prior when I'd consistently seen blood in my stool after long runs. They didn't find anything, and the doctor dismissed the blood as a result of pushing myself too hard. He said that running can cause too much impact or jarring in the bowels, which can cause bloody stool patterns. He told me his daughter was also a marathon runner and this was a somewhat common occurrence among runners. "Not to worry, you should be okay." For days after the procedure, I felt so out of it. I think the anesthesiologist administered enough medication for a three-hundred-pound man. I couldn't walk up the stairs to my house or get out of bed for three days. It felt like an angry hangover that wouldn't go away. My recollection of the colonoscopy was not a favorable one to say the least.

But this night, by this point, I was begging for the procedure. I would have done anything to stop the pain. Back in my room, I kept drifting in and out of sleep. Every time I woke up, it seemed someone new was there—nurses, doctors, shift changes—all asking the same questions, even though my chart was hanging at the foot of the bed. Each time one of them lifted the sheet, I saw him or her trying to hide an expression of horror at the size of my stomach.

"When do I go in for the colonoscopy?" I kept asking, even begging. I thought it would relieve my pain and suffering for sure. "Remove

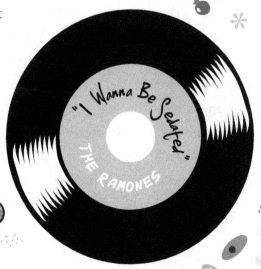

that obstruction and I'll be outta here!" I wanted to yell. Each time I asked, I was told the same thing: they were waiting on the gastroenterologist. I waited for hours. At some point, I fell asleep, and when I woke up and saw Mark, I began to get angry. "When are they going to do this damned colonoscopy, anyway?" He smiled at me and told me that I'd just awoken from the anesthesia—the test had already been done.

"You don't feel better now?" Mark asked. They'd told him that they'd found no obstruction, but he'd thought probing the area would have relieved some of the pain.

"No," I said with a big air of disgust. I still felt the same. Worse even. And my stomach was still bloated. *WTF? Why didn't it work?* There were still no answers. I was still in pain. There was no obstruction, nothing to remove as they'd initially thought. (It turns out the initial scans were read incorrectly and they weren't looking at the right side.) Back to the drawing board. It was the changing of the guard in the ER so the new docs decided to order a series of X-rays.

Since I couldn't keep anything down, they gave me iodine enemas so they could see inside me with the X-rays. Yay! More things stuck up my ass. Things just kept getting better. They wheeled me into the room and transferred me from the mobile stretcher to a stainless-steel table. A *cold* stainless-steel table. I was lying face up, bright lights beaming into my eyes, while my butt cheeks were flush up against the cold metal. It literally felt like I was freezing my ass off. When I looked up, I saw several nurses, doctors, and technicians surrounding me. All these faces, all talking to each other, about me, looking at charts, test results. I got really scared. They turned me over one way, then another. They continued to adjust my body position to get every angle. The X-ray process seemed like an eternity. I felt as though I was living an alternate reality. I was in so much pain I couldn't think clearly. The world around me seemed surreal.

After the X-rays, they brought me back to my room in the ER, where Mark was still waiting. A new doctor came in and said, "After looking at the X-rays, we aren't sure what's going on." *Glory-effing hallelujah!* I thought. While I'd been getting X-rays, they'd asked Mark if we had a surgeon, but with no explanation about why we might need one. Mark had called a friend of his, Steve, an anesthesiologist, who worked at the hospital and would have a good reference for a surgeon. In my eyes, Mark was as cool as a cucumber the entire time. He had his head on straight, unlike some of us (not mentioning any names), who almost lost it when I heard that someone we knew, in our group of friends, had been pulled into the fold. This was completely for my own good, of course. Mark had reached out to someone who could provide a reliable and highly reputable reference, someone who had years of tenure and experience in this hospital and worked with these doctors on a daily basis. Still, I was filled with anxiety.

The cat was now out of the bag, which meant my hospitalization would be up for conversation among my friends. Even during that critical moment, I was worried about what other people would think. I knew how many people were questioning my health and weight. I didn't want to fuel their fire. I could already hear the buzz about me, my "condition," and the gossip that would ensue after the word got out about my hospitalization. I would look weak, flawed, helpless. All words that were my kryptonite.

I wanted to tell Mark to make sure Steve didn't tell anyone where I was or what was happening, although I was so out of it I don't think

I was putting full sentences together. I tried to listen in as doctors updated Mark on my situation and discussed what they were planning next, though I kept falling in and out of consciousness. The next thing I recall, I was being wheeled into a private room, but then I passed out again. When I awoke, I could see out the window of my room into the hallway where six men in white coats were conversing and looking at my chart. Steve was there too. With all the pain meds flowing through my veins, I might have mistaken them for angels, but I knew better. Then I drifted off again.

Finally, later Friday afternoon, one of the doctors came in and told me they still weren't sure what was going on and that I was going to be kept overnight for observation. The overachiever in me immediately went into overdrive. I was stressing out, screaming on the inside, *This is unacceptable! I don't even understand what you're monitoring! Other than trying to manage my pain, you haven't got a clue what's causing this. I've been here almost a full day. You've done all these tests, but you have no idea what's wrong.* Irritated, exasperated, and afraid, I almost lost it as I cried to Mark: "I don't know how long I can stay here, the kids are at home . . ."

"It's okay, Ellen," Mark said. "Your mom's with the kids."

Still. It seemed like all we were doing was waiting. I had entered the hospital in the wee hours of the morning on Friday. Spring break started on Monday. My son's birthday was on Tuesday. And Wednesday, Mark and I were going to California, leaving the kids with my parents. I lost it again. Given my pain, frustration, and lack of control, I didn't hold back. There it was, that familiar voice, trying to control the situation based on my own personal agenda.

"Yeah," the doc said, "well, we're going to take you up to your room now, 807."

More waiting. Mark sat in the chair next to the bed. We were talking, the TV on in the background. I was drifting in and out. Within the hour—it was about 8:30 p.m. by that time—a guy in a white lab coat busted in, walked right up to me, and said, "Hi. My name's Dr. Michael Lindstrom. We're going to take you into surgery."

I just looked at him like, *You're who? And you're doing what?*

"We need to get going."

"What are you talking about?" I asked. "Go where?"

He went into his whole scientific dissertation about what was going on, and maybe not in exactly these words, I said, "I've been here for almost twenty-four hours, and nobody can tell me what's going on. And then, boom—you're taking me into surgery. I don't think so. Why now? What's going on?!?!?" And then I went into my whole spiel: "You've done all these tests. Nobody's told me anything. I'm here for monitoring. I'm going out of town next week. It's my son's birthday. It's spring break. Why right now? Why do you have to do it right this minute?" Blah, blah, blah.

He patiently explained again, in lay terms, what was going on. And I listened this time, trying not to panic. My colon was tied in a knot. An actual knot. As he explained this, a sense of dread filled me. The knot was stopping anything from getting into or out of me. Nothing could get through. Toxicity was building up inside me.

I had so many questions: "What kind of surgery? Can it wait? How long will I have to stay? When can I travel?" And, of course, my vanity chimed in and wanted to know if the surgery could be laparoscopic. I didn't want some big split down my middle. Because, well, bikinis. I was in full management mode, and while I was panicking, I still didn't realize the magnitude of what was happening.

I'm not sure how this had gone undetected. I still don't know, but at the time, I wasn't thinking about that. I was too frightened.

"I need to take out the blockage and repair the damage," Dr. Lindstrom said.

He told me it was a major surgery. I'd be under for at least five or six hours, and then I'd have to stay in the hospital for a week to ten days. *Holy crap! Seriously?!?* That's when things really started to sink in. When I started in with more questions and excuses again, he cut me off.

"I'm not answering your questions until you understand how dire a situation this is. You have to understand. This has to be done now. *Right now.* Your colon has been blocked for more than twenty-four hours. We don't know how much longer it will maintain this pressure. If your colon bursts, then all the toxicity that's backed up will get into your system. It's fatal. F-A-T-A-L. It can burst at any moment. At. Any. Moment."

I looked at him, speechless. I could feel a rock in my stomach. My throat closed up. There was no time to waste, none! I waved my white flag and gave up any attempt at control. The word "fatal" hit me like a brick. It finally sunk in.

"Wheel me in."

In the OR, I was surrounded by white sterile walls with bright florescent lights beaming overhead. Stainless steel tables displayed shiny metal objects lined up in an orderly fashion. They hoisted me up and transferred me to the operating table. There were about six people in the room with masks over their noses and mouths. I made eye contact with them, knowing my life was in their hands. I prayed everything would be okay.

I was in a fog. Dr. Lindstrom came toward me and reintroduced himself. Then the anesthesiologist lowered a mask over my mouth and nose. It felt like I was suffocating. I could barely breathe. He instructed me to stay calm and to slowly count backwards from the number ten. I nodded and then started, slowly . . . I was trying to breathe and count, the way I counted the miles backward as I ran: ten . . . nine . . . eight . . . seven . . . six . . .

ICU and Beyond

NEXT THING I KNEW, I woke up in the ICU. I was alive. Though I looked like an intubated ghost—tubes coming out of every place possible. Needles and IVs in the veins in my legs, arms, and both hands. A catheter. Tubes running through my nose and down my throat. I spent the first two days of my weeklong stay in the hospital in the ICU, my vitals all over the place, nurses waking me every five hours to check the machines, the needles, my safety. Often, they would panic because my blood pressure readings were so low, calling the doctor to ensure that I was not about to die. They, of course, would not take my word for it. Though I felt weak, exhausted, and had the worst case of cottonmouth I'd ever experienced, I knew I wasn't dying.

No one would give me anything to eat or drink. *Nothing! Nada! Zilch!* They said my digestive system couldn't handle it. I begged for ice chips. Begged. Finally, on the verge of tears, I got through to a young-ish ICU nurse. I told her I really needed something to drink.

She said I wasn't allowed to sip anything, but she agreed to smuggle in ice chips for me to chew on, only if I promised to take them one at a time. Let me tell you, those ice chips were my savior. Seriously, I remember thinking they were the best thing that I'd ever tasted, and I savored every moment as they melted in my mouth. I didn't get any food, at all, until my fourth day in the hospital.

And the nights. The nights were like some kind of vision quest. I felt a sense of peaceful urgency. The peace part was ironic because nights in a hospital are anything but restful—staff changes, new IVs, medications, monitors beeping, phones ringing, people being carted through the hallways on stretchers and in wheelchairs. The first night after the surgery, instead of sleeping in the wee hours, I lay in the dark, in stillness, awake and alert. So many thoughts entered my mind. I had to document them! I wanted to capture these feelings of how important it was to slow down, savor life. I was ready to release this go, go, go, miles-past-stop kind of lifestyle. I felt overwhelmed with the intense emotions emanating from deep within me. It actually felt like diarrhea of the heart. These sensations surged at me so fast and furious that I was bursting. I had never, ever, felt anything like this before, this self-love, this sense of profound purpose, this depth of gratitude.

Now, some people would say this was a normal thing—to feel so very connected to my core values, to feel so thankful for being given a second chance—but for me, it wasn't. I'm not an emotional person. But in the dark moments of those sterile hospital nights, I realized that my life up to that point had brought me to this room. I understood that the incision in my gut had opened up pathways to my brain that I had never felt before. My heart felt open to new possibilities and I was ready to chart new territory, to embrace growth. It became clear that this incision in my gut directly affected my thoughts, desires, and aspirations. Yes, my gut and my brain were in constant communication, and I could finally hear their conversation. I realized for the first time how critical it is that we listen to what our gut has to say—the butterflies, the trepidation, the intuition. They are all signals firing from the gut to the brain and back. And I really needed to listen to mine. I had to extract myself (not by choice) from my current state of being in order to gain this necessary perspective. What I realized on those nights, isolated in my hospital bed, was that the choices I had made to that point had landed me there in that room, and now it was up to me to honor and rebuild my gut and my life, and to tune in to my intuition. I knew I must slow things down to listen, whether through mindfulness, breath, or being forced to sit still. I had no other choice.

I needed to write all this down. The feelings were so intense, so I grabbed my calendar, turned to the back, and started writing. I couldn't risk forgetting what was percolating from within, the thoughts and powerful feelings bubbling up one after the other. So, high on pain meds, completely flayed open and vulnerable, I journaled for hours. It was scary. I was writing from my gut, writing from deep-seated beliefs and emotions buried under layers of dirt and filth that had overtaken my gut. I'd been cleaned out, the dust removed, and the clarity was truly brilliant. I wrote every night in the hospital, each night on a different colored page, discovering the new guiding principles in my life.

Up until that point, my treadmill had one speed—go faster. I'd never had a pause button, and so the Universe created one for me with the hospitalization. I knew that running—metaphorically or figuratively—could no longer be my fix. But I couldn't envision still-ness—ever. Quiet and solitude just weren't in my lexicon. What frightened me the most about relinquishing my running was how I would get that rush, that runner's high. That sense of worth, accomplishment, intensity, and euphoria I felt after completing a run. The constant pounding allowed me to vent my anxiety and frustration like nothing else I'd experienced. But in that room, staring at those white walls, I finally heard my gut telling me that I needed to be, just be. Doing was no longer serving me. The incision in my gut had opened both my heart and my mind.

One night, I wrote about needing to lighten my load, to stop consuming—an activity to which I applied the same determination and level of excellence I did to everything else in my life. It was time for me to stop worrying about my clothes and my house and what I needed to *buy* next. It was time for me to reduce, reuse, and recycle, to make a clean break from my old pattern of retail therapy.

My buying habits were just another way of filling my life with things that gave me a false sense of pleasure, that improved my mood and sense of self, but clouded the path I really needed to see. The fast pace of my life and these "must-have" items were all void of any real meaning. I kept hearing my second brain—my gut—during those sleepless nights. Finally, it all started to make sense. *Slow down, enjoy the scenery, stop racing, Ellen. Let your mind rest and you will regain clarity and strength.* This would help me get better. I just knew it.

Something had shifted.

This doesn't mean I did a complete 180. During the day, I vacillated, sometimes trying to step right back into the fire. I made calls from my hospital bed in an attempt to keep my life organized, letting people know I'd had emergency surgery and would be out of commission for a brief period. I called the instructor of the women's restorative yoga class I'd started three weeks prior, telling him I'd need to miss the next three to four classes, but would be back as soon as possible (even though at that point, I couldn't move a muscle). I called my clients, those I trained at my studio and others I'd taught or trained at the gym quite regularly. I spoke with Kerry, my Ayurvedic practitioner, and Rosa, my acupuncturist, who were both concerned and kind. I also called Cassie, my running coach. She expressed her concern, though it didn't feel as warm and fuzzy as the others. Her response felt more like "I'm not surprised." Some of the women in the group also called me, but I was pretty out of it, and I don't remember much about those conversations.

Mark was there every morning and every evening, sometimes during the day if I had a scheduled visit from a doctor or a follow-up with the surgeon. He was super supportive the entire time, reporting on the kids, our family, and our friends. He updated me on all the people who'd heard I was in the hospital, who wanted to bring dinner for our family, or to come by and visit. He was my connection to the outside world and showed me how very important I was to him, without any words. He brought the kids by a couple times once I was moved out of the ICU and into a hospital room. They were very into all the gadgets and monitors and the TV mounted high upon the wall. We had birthday cake for Harrison's eleventh birthday in the hospital room. And yes, I was the one who placed the order for the cake so that my son could, indeed, have candles to blow out on his birthday. Being in his presence, watching his excitement as he blew out the candles on his cake was so therapeutic for me, and for him. Celebrating his birthday in the hospital didn't seem to faze him a bit. It was truly a gift to me to be able to share in part of the celebration.

I felt loved and supported by all the people coming to see me. My parents, of course, my sister, and several of my friends, clients, and co-workers. The Rabbi and his wife came by to offer their blessings for healing. One day during visiting hours, the manager at the gym where I was teaching stopped by. When she saw that I had to have a nurse actually move my legs from one side of the bed to another, her face froze.

"Oh my G-d. Aren't you freaking out?"

I just looked at her with a blank expression, seeing for the first time just how silly it was to think in those terms.

"I mean you of all people . . .will you ever be able to run again? Look at you. Seriously, aren't you freaking out?" The last time she saw me I'd been jumping up and down like a mad woman, leading my class in an intense interval training exercise. Then, after class, I'd taken off for a run.

I didn't miss a beat. "No, I'm thankful to be alive."

She just stared at me in shock. "How can you be so calm?"

It was a natural response. Instead of dwelling on the events of the recent past, I was so focused on the present moment, and—for once—not worried, anxious, or freaked out about my future. I was looking within and could finally hear the quiet beat of my own heart. The me who had been in constant motion and constant flux was finally still, and I could hear.

"I'm just happy to be here, really," I said. "Things could have been so much worse. If they hadn't caught this in time, I would have died.

I'm so fortunate things turned out as they did, to be in this space. Right here, right now. This is truly a blessing."

I continued to believe that after I was released from the hospital, I would no longer quiet my newly recognized "gut voice." I wouldn't drown it out with the noise I had created before. Even though I was afraid, and didn't know how to be still, as long as I listened to my gut, I felt I would find a way. I was never going back to the person that almost did me in. I swore to myself that I would hold on to this newfound awareness, embrace it, live by it.

Five days after the surgery, they released me from the hospital. I was originally told that my stay would be seven to ten days, so I was excited to have been granted an early exit. I was officially on the road to recovery. I went to see Rosa not long after I got out of the hospital, and she told me to focus on this feeling of peacefulness, serenity, and gratitude. Remember it, live it each and every day. Because, if I didn't, my former persona was strong and powerful, and I could easily resort to my familiar habits. I didn't believe her. I would not believe her.

But each and every day, I got stronger. The previous me kept trying to creep back in, trying to get me to start my frenetic race again. As I began to feel more alive and wean myself from the pain meds,

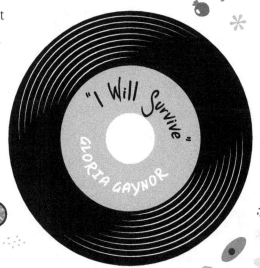

I dug deep for that hard-wired strength and determination to help me heal.

It felt as if I had a bad guy on one shoulder whispering to me that I should start running again. He took over, furiously, shoving my new calm, serene self out. The good guy, on my other shoulder, told me to rest, to be enough, that I *was* enough. The bad guy kept yelling louder and louder in my ear, screaming at me to race again.

Soon, no longer vulnerable, in pain, and alone in my hospital room, I began dismissing everything the doctors had told me not to do. After two weeks at home, I walked outside to get the mail. I felt the same sensation, almost, as when I completed my first marathon. It was a feeling of overwhelm, delight, pride, and accomplishment. Next I began walking the dog. Then walking around the large circle I lived on, to the end of the street and back around again (about thirty houses), without stopping. The doctors told me I couldn't teach or train for a couple months, yet after about five weeks, I reached out to my clients, telling them to come to my studio. They could work out. I would tell them what to do. Yes, I picked up the weights. Yes, I put them back on the shelf. I moved equipment around. I was feeling better. I silently told myself it was okay, because I wasn't exercising myself. My good little guy tried to tell me, *You don't need to teach right now. You need to heal.* But the bad guy side was kicking ass.

The walk to the end of the street and around my circle was easy now. I needed a bigger challenge. The walk slowly morphed into a jog/walk, then a jog, then a run/walk, and then running became my new challenge. Each time I ran, I added a little distance. The same mentality took over. *Just a little more. Just a little more.* There was no question the bad guy had taken the lead and the good guy was completely out of sight.

After about a month or so of this running/walking routine, I called Cassie to tell her I was ready to start running with the group again. I felt nervous, uneasy because of the intervention, and because of the response I received on the other end of the line when I'd called her from the hospital. I didn't tell my family I was going to start up with the group again. So when I called, I called from inside our bedroom closet, where I sometimes went when everyone was at home and I wanted to have a private moment.

I sat on the floor of my closet, doors closed, heart racing, every insecurity I possessed rising to the surface: *What did Cassie think of me? Well, I have a pretty good idea. And what about the others in the group? Did they feel the same way? Did they lose all faith in their friend? Did they think that my actions had landed me on that operating table?* There was trepidation about running with them again, but I also felt the excitement brewing. I longed for the warmth and comradery of the group.

"Hi, it's Ellen," I said when Cassie answered. "I wanted to speak to you about coming back to running group."

"No," she said. "I can't have you back. You can't come back. It's too much."

"What?" *She must mean not quite yet.*

"I'm worried. I'm concerned for you. You know our workouts are very intense. For all I know, you could keel over and die any second. You should not be doing them. I won't have you. It's too much pressure on me and I don't want that liability. I don't think it's the right thing for either of us."

I was shocked. This is not what I had expected to hear. I started crying, sobbing. "Cassie, please." I couldn't even fathom not going back. These women were my rock. I had felt as if everything else had been pulled out from under me, but not this. Noooooo, not this too!

"No. I'm not letting you come back. Even when you get better and you're strong—"

"But I *am* better. Now."

"I don't think you are. I don't think you're healed."

"I am. I swear I am. I . . ." I couldn't finish. I was crying too hard.

"You said that after lunch, then you ended up in the hospital."

I begged, I pleaded between huge gulping sobs. "Cassie, please. I'm better. It wasn't the running that landed me in the hospital. My colon was tied in a knot. I can run again. And I promise not to push too hard. I promise!"

But she wouldn't budge. She didn't want the liability or the baggage. She didn't believe I was strong enough mentally or physically to come back, and nothing I said or did was going to convince her otherwise. I sat in that closet long after we hung up, filled with too much shame to open the doors. Shame and a devastating sense of loss. I yearned for the comfort and support I received from those women. And I needed them now more than ever. Partially, I craved the workouts. But mainly, I felt I was being torn from this group of women who had been my lifeline.

Running was the glue that connected me to them. It was my weekly sanctuary, my church. I knew I probably wouldn't see them anymore. And even if I did, I'd be too ashamed to speak to them. They would have heard the whole story from Cassie about my total and complete breakdown when I heard I could no longer be a part of the group. They'd probably think it was all about the intensity, the training, the race prep, but it wasn't that at all. I needed them, I needed their strength, their levelheadedness, their accountability.

Dr. Lindstrom had saved my life. Had I been firing on all cylinders, I would have seen the surgery as my Universal Intervention, kind of like three strikes and you're out. But, I wasn't out. I was alive and still in the game. This third and final wake-up call was a message to get my exercise addiction and disordered eating under control. It was time to shit or get off the pot.

Kripalu

BACK IN THE FALL, way before the surgery, when Kerry and I had been meeting on a regular basis, we'd discussed my desire to escape for a while. She suggested I go on a retreat and disconnect from the everyday hustle and bustle of life. I agreed that it was time for a big honkin' reset. An escape or distraction from my everyday routine was exactly what I needed in order to embrace what both Kerry and Rosa urged me to do—stop, breathe, and ground. Kerry offered a few options, though we both knew an ashram was a little too extreme for me. I wanted to continue immersing myself in the study of Ayurveda and learn its guiding principles and history. I had a desire to learn more about how this information applied to me and my health. Kerry suggested Kripalu Center for Yoga & Health in Massachusetts.

I read through Kripalu's website and clicked on the tab under "School of Ayurveda." This was it! It felt like a perfect fit.

I ran it by Rosa at my next appointment and she was totally on board. I spoke to Mark about going to this program in the spring as a belated birthday gift and he was amenable, so within a few days, my trip was booked! I put it in my calendar and started counting down the days. Six months seemed like an eternity, especially since I was looking forward to it with so much excitement and anticipation.

I would often hear, *I'm going to Kripalu, I'm going, I'm going,* in the back of my mind, especially when I needed a little extra lift or oomph in my day. So, as you can imagine, one of the first questions I had after regaining consciousness from my surgery was, "Can I still go to Kripalu in April?" The answer was "Yes, you should be fine to go, Ellen."

In that month between leaving the hospital and heading to Kripalu, my life became a minefield of constantly shifting perceptions. I'd have a moment of clarity (*Don't go there again. Let up a little. Loosen the reins.*), immediately followed by intense panic (*How do I slow down? STFU! I am not doing as much as I used to do, promise!*), then I'd slide into denial, convincing myself I was fine (*I'm getting stronger every day. I'm feeling much better*). Always trying to outrun the hurt, the fear, and the shame.

But anytime I felt uncertain, panicked, or overwhelmed, knowing the week-long Ayurveda intensive at Kripalu was on the horizon provided some relief. Before I knew it, April had arrived and I was counting the days until my departure. I needed this now more than ever. The surgery had escalated my desire to escape, reset, and delve deeper into the study of Ayurveda to discover what else would be revealed to me about my healing. "I'm going" quickly became "I'm here."

When I arrived at the retreat in Stockbridge, Massachusetts, I felt so happy, so free. It was absolutely beautiful—snow-covered hills, woods, a lake. So peaceful. I couldn't remember the last time I'd taken time out for myself for any extended period. I checked in at the reception desk. They handed me a packet containing a map of the grounds, the main highlights, and the areas I would be frequenting most often throughout my stay, including the building where my room was located. I'd chosen a single. This was, in essence, a retreat, and I needed time alone, completely alone, to reset and recharge.

My room was smallish, with white walls, a bed with crisp, white sheets, a bureau, a bathroom with a sink and shower, and a lamp on the nightstand. It was simple and very serene. Just standing there and taking in this private space relaxed me. There were no electronics, not even a digital alarm clock by the bed. All the amenities were green and sustainable; the building was as well. The towels were made of soft, organic cotton. There were cards in the room asking guests to please use the water sparingly, reuse towels, and recycle. The room smelled clean and fresh, not at all like chemicals, but more like crisp linens. I looked out the window and saw a labyrinth, the lake, and beautiful trees with their branches still bare. My pulse began to slow down. I exhaled and felt a sense of calm come over my body. It was getting late so I made my way to the dining hall, had some dinner, and returned to my room, exhausted from the travel but excited to start the program the next day.

The next morning, I ate breakfast in the dining hall. The buffet was filled with grains, vegetables, seaweeds, oatmeal, various nut milks, fresh fruit, seeds, nuts, eggs, pancakes, raw honey, hot tea. There were so many options. Everything looked delicious and so very fresh. After a beautiful and satisfying breakfast, I headed over to the next building to start my Ayurvedic immersion. In the classroom, which had no tables, chairs, or desks, we all gathered on the floor in one big circle. Meditation cushions and blankets softened our seats. Windows surrounded the room, offering a panoramic view of the grounds.

There were thirty of us in the class. We introduced ourselves and offered some insight about what had brought us there. When it was my turn, I said, "I've been working with an Ayurvedic practitioner in Austin for about nine months. I learned about the doshas and recognized how my dosha combination mirrored me, my personality, and my lifestyle so perfectly. I discovered how the principles of the science help rebalance the doshas and wanted to learn more." I told them I'd signed up several months ago and had been looking forward to coming, though about a month earlier, I'd had major surgery and almost died. "My colon was tied in a knot." Telling a group of thirty strangers that I'd almost died a month ago felt scary and awkward and real. I was a little nervous to put it all out there, but then I thought, *If not now, when?*

"I've been searching for answers about my health for a *long* time," I said, "and when I found Ayurveda, I embraced the principles. It all made so much sense—the lifestyle, the eating, the calming modalities, the bodywork. That's why I'm here. I want to learn as much as I can about how to apply these principles to myself, how to embrace these changes, and how to help others understand themselves through the eyes of Ayurveda."

That first day, we also met the staff who would be working with us as well as some students who were enrolled in the School of Ayurveda at Kripalu. We learned about the history of Ayurveda, got a very detailed explanation of each of the doshas, and then took a short quiz to classify ourselves in one or a combination of them. For the rest of the course, we went on to study all aspects of Ayurveda. We spent a day in the kitchen learning about the foods and cooking methods. We learned about the doshas of the mind: *Satvic* (focused, calm, imparts balance, free from attachment), *Rajasic* (passionate, never satisfied, many attachments), and *Temasek* (dull, heavy, impulsive), and the foods that promote a balance among the three. We spoke a lot about our imbalances and did exercises to identify them, prioritize them, and strategize how to bring ourselves closer to equanimity.

During our free time, we were encouraged to experience some of the Ayurvedic bodywork that Kripalu offered. There were so many options. I wish I could have tried them all. I opted for the Abhyanga massage, which uses a customized oil blend to balance and rejuvenate your constitution, and rhythmic strokes to help the energy flow through the body and relax the nerves. I also experienced *Shirodhara*, a soothing treatment where a constant flow of oil is dripped on your forehead, over your third eye. It's incredibly calming to the mind, body, and spirit, enhancing blood circulation in your brain and helping to relieve stress and tension. Seriously, I don't think I've ever felt more relaxed in my life.

We ate in a dining hall that offered macrobiotic, vegetarian and vegan selections, a sandwich bar, and a Buddha Bar offering very simple grains, vegetables, and broths. I was overwhelmed and delighted by all the good, clean, healthy food I didn't have to prepare myself. I can't say Mark and the kids would have been so thrilled with these offerings, but I thought I had entered foodie heaven on earth. The bright display of seasonal organic vegetables, the seaweed, the vegan soups, the herbal teas; even the desserts were clean and healthy.

One day, one of our assignments was to eat all of our meals in silence. Of course, the first thing I did after fixing my breakfast plate and sitting down with some people from my group was to greet them with a big friendly "Good morning!" They just stared at me with big eyes, and I got it. *Oops, I fucked that one up right from the get go.* I was kind of embarrassed and, at first, tempted to leave and head over to the dining room where people ate in absolute silence. Yep, they have a separate room for that. I noticed people in there every day, but they didn't really seem like "my people." Some looked very contemplative, Zen, dressed in all-white scarves and tunics. They were focused, grounded, in a meditative state. I was curious to know if they always ate in silence, even when they weren't at Kripalu? Even if they didn't, I couldn't relate. I just preferred to stay in the larger area where everyone seemed to be more my speed.

In one of our discussions, we were told that chewing every mouthful of food promotes better digestion and keeps us focused on our meal. The food should be an even consistency prior to swallowing. Foods not chewed properly may lead to gas, bloating, and fermentation. Boy, did this information hit home! Bingo! Another interesting point we learned about eating was that you actually burp when your body is satiated. It takes a little while for the food to digest before your body feels satisfied. If you listen, you will hear it. Every. Single. Time. But our culture is so accustomed to eating on the run, in front of screens, while texting, driving, and listening to loud music—sometimes all at the same time—we never even know it's occurred. We pay absolutely no attention to what we eat, how fast we eat it, the tastes, smells, textures. We inhale food and eat mindlessly, not chewing, not listening to our bodies. We are distracted eaters. Our teachers told us to listen for the burp. So, in my silence, I listened. And, yes, there it was, loud and clear as day. I was amazed at how simple it was to read my body's signals and interpret exactly how it was feeling. I was starting to recognize the benefits of being more present, paying attention to the details, quieting my mind and my body.

Every night, we practiced *Yoga Nidra*, a deep relaxation technique. We would lie on our yoga mats and the facilitator would take us on a guided meditative journey. Immediately afterward, I would head back to my room and write down all the thoughts I'd had and insights I'd gained during this peaceful exercise. One night, I had to call Mark to tell him about my experience, it was so profound. I read the following passage to him:

I stated my intention: To continue healing myself by listening to the signs my body is giving me.

The facilitator guided us on a journey through a door, across a grassy field filled with flowers. The first flower I saw was a yellow wildflower. I also saw red Indian paintbrush, bluebonnets, dandelions, and many Black-eyed Susans.

We were then directed to go through a gate. There was a symbol on the gate. At first, I just saw white iron with an ornate design, but then I saw a lotus flower. The gate opened and I was traveling down a gravel path through a forest filled with pine trees. I observed at the end of this path the oldest, most established tree in the forest. I noticed the bark, needles, branches, and trunk. My eyes traveled down the trunk until I saw its roots. I noticed where the roots entered the earth, then looked down into the earth, where the roots had established themselves underground.

At the base of the tree, the roots had tied themselves into a knot. The facilitator told us to think of a color. I didn't really see a color clearly, but I thought of yellow.

I pictured yellow in my mind's eye and visualized the small yellow wildflower I'd seen earlier in the field. The facilitator told us to visualize a symbol. As I began to see the small yellow wildflower appear, the image of a yellow sunflower began to emerge. As she spoke about the symbol, I began to see the details of the sunflower materialize. Its leaves were yellow and its center was brown. It had a thick stalk. I then pictured the vase filled with sunflowers that had been on the altar at the front of our classroom all week. I realized this was symbolic of the changes that were happening at Kripalu. I began to think about the sunflower oil I'd been told was good for my dosha, denoting its nourishing properties. I thought of the sunflower seeds on the bar in the dining hall symbolizing the proper foods I should be eating to bring my dosha into balance.

As the vision ended, I saw a big bouquet of yellow sunflowers in an arrangement on my kitchen table. I thought about asking Mark to buy some sunflowers to greet me upon my return.

I've felt a change coming on for some time, but everything seemed to gel here. I need to be sure, certain, and determined to maintain my focus and listen to my body, my inner voice, upon my return to Austin.

I'm thankful to my teachers for giving me this information, my practitioners at home who have helped me heal and will continue to assist me as I move forward. I'm especially thankful for my village of family and friends who, out of genuine love for me and my

health, have guided, supported, assisted, intervened, and questioned
me through this process.

I'm blessed to have been given this opportunity, this gift. I
want to pass my knowledge and wisdom on to others.

I have enjoyed several years of teaching classes and training
wonderful individuals. Now it's time for me to take a step back in
the physical realm of exercise and allow my body to heal. When
I'm physically healthier, I want to continue to learn about the age-
old science of Ayurveda. My desire is to bring its teachings back
to the community that has entrusted me for so long and educate
them more holistically about how to improve their health.

I've finally found the last piece of the puzzle for which I've
been searching. Namaste.

When I finished reading, Mark was quiet. I could feel he also
believed a shift was occurring. We said "I love you," then I hung up
the phone and drifted off to sleep.

One afternoon, we had some free time and I booked an appointment with the head of the School of Ayurveda, Rosie, to gain more
insight into myself and my dosha. Just as Kerry had, she pegged me
immediately, and offered more of the same advice I'd been receiving
but not listening to: "You're very Vata," she said. "*Very* Vata." She
repeated much of what Kerry had told me. She also suggested that I
cook with coconut oil at least three times per week. She talked about
the importance of spices. She told me to simmer cumin and fennel
seeds for two to three minutes and drink the tea to calm my *agni*,
or digestive fire, and increase the absorption of my food. Another
suggestion was to incorporate the herbs *asafoetida* and *ashwaganda*

to help pacify my Vata and help my compromised digestion. "You need to ground yourself. Get more Kapha." As she talked, I nodded. "Okay. Okay." I was taking copious notes and this time, I was on it. Her words were sinking in. I was finally resonating with advice I had been ignoring for years.

On the very first day of the retreat, we were encouraged to use the week to relax, take it easy. If we were going to do anything active, it should be done without much exertion (read, walk around the Labyrinth and conduct a walking meditation, go to a restorative yoga class, do some breathing exercises). I felt very relaxed the first couple of days I was there. I was able to unwind and immerse myself in some of the bodywork, explore the campus and outdoors a little bit. I took a yoga class. But by the end of the second day, I had ants-in-my-pants from sitting all day, not exercising (yoga was nothing too strenuous), and from the anxiety-driven fear that slowing down brings to a consciousness unaccustomed to decelerating. Afraid I would lose the fitness I'd struggled to regain, I craved intensity and needed to get my fix. While the experiences there were wonderful, I wasn't able to completely let go.

So in the early morning hours of my third day at Kripalu, I awoke as the sun peeked through the blinds. But instead of meditating, going to yoga, and then chewing forever before class started at 9:00, as we were instructed to do, I headed over to the gym. A very *tiny* gym. Kripalu has several large spaces for practicing yoga, dance, and meditation, but their gym (for the hundreds of people there) was the size of a bedroom. I stood in the door, taking in the few stability balls, weights, mats, an elliptical, and the one treadmill in the corner, which didn't look like it got much use. Without hesitation, I jumped on and proceeded to run six miles, eyes glued to the odometer, my favorite playlist blasting from my iPod. I was back in my zone. It was too cold for me to do anything outside, so unbeknownst to anyone else in my program, I opted to start my day on the treadmill for those next few mornings.

I felt like I was cheating everyone by breaking protocol, but I was actually cheating myself. I felt the tug from both directions—ashamed that I was probably the only one in the group who couldn't follow the recommended guidelines, but also needing to fulfill my craving for intensity and quash any fear of letting go. So I ran. After my runs, I'd bolt back to my room to shower, then quickly eat breakfast before class started. I certainly didn't chew my food appropriately or relax as I was eating. I was pressed for time, which made me anxious.

Despite the suggestion to not overexert ourselves, I told myself it was okay to run. In my mind, this was loosely interpreted as *It's okay if I run just a few miles.* As I ran, I heard Rosie's words in my mind about creating too much wind energy, but I was addicted. To start my day with a clear mind, to relieve any anxiety, and absolve any fear of not holding onto my level of fitness, I ran. Nothing

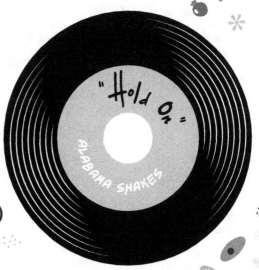

111

could relax me like running. It was that feeling of accomplishment after the run that I craved, that euphoric release of endorphins. Still, each and every time I started, I felt anxious, knowing both the mental and physical struggle that lay ahead. My body was going to reject the impact and intensity, though I couldn't allow my mind to back down. I felt guilty (a little) and upset with myself (a lot) that I couldn't embrace the environment, the experience, and the solitude that I had craved for so long. I wouldn't listen to the very people I sought out to teach me and counsel me on what I so desperately wanted to learn. I was being pulled by that bad guy on my shoulder and knew it, though I didn't have the strength, the willpower, or the tenacity to stand up to him . . . yet.

On the final day of the retreat, we spent the entire time discussing what it would be like when we returned to our everyday, overbooked, plugged in, Starbucks-fueled lives (did I mention that caffeine was a big no-no too?). As the group shared the realities of returning to their real lives—kids, no coffee, work, homes, social media, a gazillion commitments, no coffee—anxiety filled the room.

We were all freaking out. How could we hold onto this amazing feeling we'd been immersed in for the last several days? How could we incorporate all that we were supposed to do—eight hours of sleep, scrape our tongues, dry brush our skin, Abhyanga massage—when we had to make lunches; get kids dressed, fed, and off to school; fight traffic; run errands; keep our houses clean; pick up kids; deliver them to games and after-school activities; work a forty-hour work week (for some); make dinner . . . *Please!*

"You realize that you're going to be reintegrating into your real world and that some of these things are going to have to fall off," our teacher said in a very calm, respectful voice. "It's absolutely normal and natural. You'll have to experiment with them a little bit then see what sticks. The things that are most helpful for you are the things that I would focus on when creating your routine. What's been the most effective? What's changed you the most while you've been here? Can you make time to meditate in the morning? Is it easier to meditate at night? Where will you meditate? Can you create a sanctuary all your own? Are you going to practice Yoga Nidra? Will you get a CD and listen to Jennifer's voice as you did here just a few evenings ago?"

I was scared shitless. Seriously. We all were. Reintegration would be difficult and letting go was inevitable. We wanted to hold onto everything, but the reality was that many of our experiences from Kripalu would just disappear into thin air. We couldn't live at Kripalu. The instructor suggested we create a schedule to follow, and no one had to tell my Type-A personality twice. I got right on it during my flight back to Austin, spending several hours charting and laying out my schedule, not only to the minute, but to the thirty seconds.

My Pitta, in all its glory, went to work. The entire flight I drafted a schedule on paper spread out on my tiny tray, trying to make perfect lines representing the divisions of days in the week as the plane bumped over the wind pockets. I was already getting annoyed. I began filling in blocks of time, assigning each rectangle with an hour of the day, revising activities so I would somehow be able to fit it all in. Over and over again until it looked, well, perfect.

If I got up at 6:00 a.m., peed/pooped, washed my face, brushed my teeth, and got dressed by 6:35, then I could eat by 6:45, get the kids in the car and off to school by 7:00. Then, after I got back home and ran, which I wasn't supposed to do, I'd shower and work in my *Abhyanga* massage, dry brushing, and tongue scraping. I needed to cook and eat lunch, prepare dinner. What would I cook for dinner? I filled in the meals for each day of the week; having a menu left nothing to chance. The entire process of hyper-planning completely stressed me out. *I'm not going to be able to do this. How can I possibly stick to all of this?* The schedule had to work. I had to follow it perfectly. Not doing so would mean I had failed and that my Ayurveda intensive at Kripalu was all for nothing. This was the complete antithesis of what I was supposed to have learned during the past week.

We were supposed to leave calmer, more grounded, balanced, with a better understanding of the things we create in our lives that throw us off kilter. Now we had the tools to return to equilibrium. Not one teacher had placed any expectation upon us to continue to live our Kripalu lives once we integrated back into our realities. I don't really think any one of the thirty people in my group expected to hold onto all these experiences either. Well, except for one. That really anal girl from Texas.

When I landed back in Austin, I was so excited to see my kids and Mark. The minute the cab dropped me off at home, I opened my front door and grabbed them in a big group hug. Then immediately it hit me: *Oh my G-d. I'm so freaking stressed out right now. How the flippin' fuck is this going to happen? How am I going to be able to be a mom and a wife and stay all Om with my Ayurveda stuff?* All of a sudden, shit got really real. But come hell or high water, I was going to try to stick to my plan.

That first night, I came into the bedroom at ten o'clock, an hour earlier than usual. Mark was already in bed.

"I'm going to bed early," I said.

"That's great," Mark said. He was trying to be completely support-ive, allowing me to incorporate what I'd learned.

"Yeah," I said, "I need to be asleep by 10:30." Thirty minutes to brush my teeth, do my whole routine with the rose water and *Nasya* oil, plug in my earphones, listen to my *Yoga Nidra* CD, write down my thoughts. Shit. It was going to be tight. I could feel my blood pressure jump up a notch. I hurried into the bathroom to get started. Then I heard the TV through the door.

I ran into the bedroom. Mark was watching the news, which we did every night. I marched over to the armoire, shut off the TV, and closed and locked the doors.

"What's up?" Mark asked.

"No wathig TV bow," I said with my mouth full of toothpaste. "Can't be on wufowre bed. Too stimulating."

"Okay." He shrugged. "You're the one who always wants it on."

"Whatever," I muttered as I ran back to the bathroom. There was no time to argue. When I finished my routine, and came back into the room, Mark was already asleep. The room had to be pitch black, so I made sure the shades were pulled down all the way, turned the clock toward the wall, and switched off the light. There was so much stuff to do!

I tasked Mark with waking up the kids, making sure they were dressed, and getting breakfast together. Each morning I went through my thirty- to forty-minute routine: washing my face, brushing my teeth, scraping my tongue, dry brushing, and Abhyangaing my entire body (which I was really supposed to do after my shower, but I didn't take a shower first thing in the morning because I worked out first [which I wasn't supposed to do], and I wouldn't have time for the entire routine later, so I had to fit it in when I got out of bed).

After about a week, Mark was getting somewhat frustrated that he was taking on most of the morning routine without any help. He didn't have time to get his swim in before work. That was his deal—he swam with a group in the mornings a few days a week before heading to the office. Always has and probably always will. My issue was that I couldn't get up an hour earlier to fit in my list of morning activities because then I wouldn't be able to get in my requisite eight hours of sleep. Ten o'clock was the earliest I could get to bed, for sure. I've always been kind of a night owl. My stress level skyrocketed—I thought I might as well throw everything I'd just learned out the window. All I could think was: *You're such a flipping failure because you can't do this. Why can't you make it all work? I bet everyone else is at home in a state of kumbaya, living, eating, and breathing everything they learned at Kripalu. Why is it so difficult for you?* I honestly had no idea if anybody else was successful or was even trying to make these things work. For all I knew, they were sitting at Starbucks sipping their venti lattes and nibbling chocolate chip muffins while checking their Facebook feeds. All that mattered was that I was failing.

Sometimes I'd just say to myself, *I need to take care of me first, because if I do this for myself, I will be a better*_____ (fill in the blank). But I wasn't really taking care of myself at all. My head went straight to: *Do it. Do it right. Do it in its entirety or else you're a loser* mentality. I was so rigid, creating such an impossible reality for myself and those who loved and supported me. I felt lost. Drifting somewhere between the desire to hold on and the desire to let it all go. Those moments of peace and clarity that appeared at Kripalu gradually faded away to barely a memory.

Finish Line

THE RACE WAS ON. I was running in the Napa to Sonoma half marathon in July, six months after surgery. Don't ask me what I was thinking, because, clearly, I wasn't. Noel and I had had our eyes on this race for more than a year. It was a tough race to get into, always sold out, so the previous December, we'd schemed and entered the minute the sign-up link went live, and we got in. Two entries into a half marathon through the wine country—check. The girls would run, and the following day, we'd tour several boutique wineries in the area with our husbands. Noel and I had been researching wineries, coordinating with drivers, and planning schedules for months. I'd booked the hotel and made plane reservations. I was committed to going. I wanted to do it. And believed I could, even if I had to make some modifications. Just train and get through the pain.

"I can do it," I told Noel.

"Sure you can," she said. "No worries. You're strong. I know you can do it. I know you." Noel is the nicest person you'll ever meet. It wouldn't occur to her not to support my decision. So I thought, *If she's encouraging me to do it, then I guess there's nothing to worry about.* Mark wasn't quite so supportive. "You're not running that race," he said.

"Of course I am. I got in. I paid for it. I'm going. All four of us are going."

Mark and I went back and forth for two weeks, then he gave up. He knew it was useless to argue with me because I'd just argue right back: "I don't know what you're talking about," or "It's just a half. I can get back to that," or "I'm fine, Mark. You don't know."

But I thought Noel knew. I love Noel dearly. We met at Pure Austin gym back in 2007, where we attended the same group workout classes, the long ones on Saturdays and Sundays, packed with weekend warriors—those who craved intensity, who pushed themselves to their max, who attended multiple classes in one day. After class one day, we got to talking and discovered we were both doing the Marble Falls Triathlon. We just clicked. As an athlete, she pushes herself as hard as I do—harder, actually. She's like the freaking Energizer Bunny—constantly exercising and perpetually researching and entering new races, triathlons, Half Ironmans, marathons, ultramarathons, overnight relays. There's always something on the horizon. From that one conversation we had after class at the gym, we became great friends. We shared a common thread: running, racing, and competing. And we were both driven, intense, committed, and strong.

Although these similarities drew us together, we led very different lives. She was a corporate executive who worked for a large Austin-based tech company. She didn't have kids. Her engineer brain thinks through things in a very calculated manner. This showed every time we ran. She'd plug our route into her watch, and at the end of our workout, she'd have the stats: her heart rate, our average pace, total distance, elevation, and calories burned. Then she'd go home and download all this information into an app. I, on the other hand, tried to tune out the beeping of her watch signaling that we had completed another mile. I didn't want to know our pace or which mile we were on because that's all I would think about until I heard it again.

We started running together every Sunday, preparing for the many races we had entered. Those Sunday runs lasted for several years. Over hundreds, maybe even thousands of miles, we learned so much about each other; we had some really deep conversations, about everything from work to workouts, from friendship to food, from spouses and siblings to sick parents—nothing was off-limits. I totally trusted her and she trusted me. The one thing that always amazed me, no matter what race we were training for, no matter what the situation, she always seemed so casual, relaxed, and care-free. She's the happy-go-lucky, totally laid-back persona and I'm the "Shit, I'm stressing, I have to do well, run harder, train more, up my game and PR" kinda gal.

When Noel competes, she does well, but she doesn't possess that intense triathlete personality—so Type-A, focused, freaking out 24/7 about every little thing from the weather to nutrition to how many ounces the bike weighs. Noel talks about exercise, but in a very light-hearted, relaxed fashion. Once she told me that she'd entered the lottery for the Kona Ironman in Hawaii. I was like, "What?! Seriously, girlfriend? What if you get in?!" She kind of chuckled, the way she often does, and said, "Well, I guess I'll just train for it."

Kona is the ultimate triathlon. It's the Ironman World Championship. You have to qualify to compete in the race. It's the best of the best of each age group in the WORLD. The Big Kahuna of all Ironmans. Intimidating for sure, but not to Noel. She wanted to run with the best of 'em. They offer a handful of slots that are open to the lottery. You can apply (with certain qualifications, of course) and those who are lucky enough get in. Well, the next trip I planned with Noel would definitely be to Las Vegas 'cause that girl got her ass in!

When Noel told me, she was like, "Guess what?" and I knew exactly what she was going to say. My stomach got all nervous for her right away. She, however, couldn't have been more excited. Maybe she said she was a little nervous because she would need to get a training plan or a coach or a something, though it was totally in jest. She was truly beside herself with joy that she would be able to race in Kona. I'd constantly wonder: *How is she doing this? How is she continually competing and running and doing these triathlons with such joy, such pleasure, and such excitement while remaining so relaxed?* I wished I could have her attitude.

Noel's presence calmed me down. I loved her faith in me. And she was so accepting, even when I needed a harder line. One Sunday, around the time of the interventions, I asked her, "Would you consider me too thin?"

She just looked at me. "No, why?"

"You know, you can tell me. Do you think I'm too skinny?"

"I think you've lost weight, but I wouldn't consider you too skinny. Why?"

"Because recently I've been getting a lot of commentary about my weight. A lot of people think I'm too thin. The running group said something. My parents said something. Mark mentioned that other people are talking about it. It's starting to get to me. It's hurtful that I'm hearing these rumblings of discussion about me and my weight behind my back. I know you would tell me if you thought otherwise, right? If you don't think I'm too thin, that's good to know. You've been running with me for all these years, so you see me every week . . ."

We were quiet for a minute. "Do you think I run too much?"

"What? No. You don't run too much."

Of course she didn't think I ran too much. She ran just as much. Even more, much more. I knew she would think it was a silly question.

After my surgery, Noel and I had to take a hiatus from our weekly runs, but after Kripalu, I called to tell her I was ready to run together again. I knew my limits—although I pushed myself to them every time. I warned her to be fair and square: "You might not want to train for the half marathon with me. I'll have to go really, really, really slowly. And I'll probably have to stop, and I probably have to Galloway." Galloway is a method where you select a run-to-walk ratio so your heart rate doesn't continue to elevate and you can maintain your stamina to finish the race without hitting the (dreaded) wall.

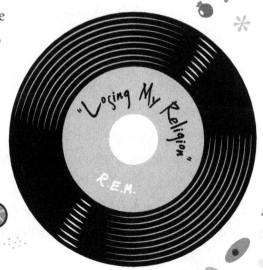

But my patient friend was just fine with moving at my pace. "Oh, yes. I'm training with you. For sure we can go slower. No worries." So off we went. Each time we ran, I'd have to make a pit stop. Sometimes two, and on a not so very good day, three. Her easygoing demeanor was not disrupted when I had to detour for a dump. Not only did Noel create and map out run courses so we could achieve our allotted training distance, she would also cleverly navigate us to the closest restroom when I was jonesin' for the john so I could make it there as quickly as possible. Once we arrived at the public potty of choice (usually a grocery store, convenience store, or coffee shop), I would bee line to the bathroom, barely making it to the toilet. Noel, if she had to pee, would always say, "I'll meet you outside when you're done." I suppose she could have done her week's grocery shopping during some of these bathroom diversions, but never, ever, did she question me or seem upset in the least about pausing her workout for the next assquake.

After I'd emerge, we'd usually walk a bit until my body could handle the jarring of the pavement again. As soon as I'd break into a light jog, she'd join in, and we'd continue to gain speed, returning to our pace until the next time my insides started rumbling. We maintained this pattern for a few months until Napa to Sonoma was upon us.

The night before the race I didn't sleep much. I didn't feel well, and felt even worse the next morning. My stomach was in knots, my head hurt, and I must have gone to the bathroom ten times in an hour attempting to eliminate everything from my system. Nerves definitely played a large part, although I was convinced the previous night's dinner also played a role. I thought maybe I'd been "glutened" or had eaten something that didn't agree with me, even though I was extremely careful about what I consumed. I fumbled around the hotel room, trying not to awaken Mark, put my race gear in my bag, made a final bathroom visit, and met Noel in the lobby.

Before we started, Noel asked me how I was feeling and if I wanted to do Galloway or just run the entire time. You can't start Galloway halfway through a race. Even if you are so pumped with adrenaline and have all the energy in the world at the start, you must start the Galloway method at the beginning, or else it just doesn't work. We both knew that.

"I can run," I told her. "I want to run."

When we arrived, there were tons of people, mostly in good spirits, awaiting the start of the race. It was beautiful, lots of greenery, wide open fields, cooler temps. Before I knew it, the gun blasted and we were on our way. We began slowly, and then got into our rhythm. The first four or five miles were relatively flat, some rolling hills but nothing too terrible. We talked and took in the beautiful weather and the vineyards around us. I kept listening for Noel's beeps from her watch. While I hated the beeps during our training runs, in a race they provided a mental check after each mile. One mile closer to the finish. Around mile six, I started to feel some pressure in my belly. This was about the time that I would normally start to feel it, so I had a feeling I'd have to use the porta-potties in the next mile or two. While I was scouting the sides of the road for the next round of blue and green plastic toilets, Noel was admiring the rolling hills and acres of grapes growing just a few feet away.

"What types of grapes do you think those are?" she asked. "Look at how these clumps of grapes differ from the ones at the vineyard we just passed. Did you see that bird? What kind do you think that was? The trees here are amazing! We don't have trees like that in Austin."

What? Huh? Clearly, I had no idea what she was saying. I looked over, nodded my head to acknowledge the grapes, the birds, and whatever else she was rambling about. All I could focus on was the increasing pressure inside me, and searching farther down the road for my big blue BFFs to show up. The cramps were coming on. Around mile seven, I spotted the toilets in the distance, picked up my pace, and ran straight to the first open porta-potty. I waved back to Noel to show her where I was headed. I took a deep breath of fresh air, opened the door, then did my best not to inhale until I exited. Since I'm a bit of a germaphobe, the porta-potty is not my ideal throne. There was no freakin' way I would actually sit, not even with three layers of TP covering the seat. I did my best in the squatty position and bailed before I needed to inhale. Once outside, I caught a glimpse of Noel, headed her way, and down the road we traveled.

Things didn't go so well after that. The cramps dissipated a bit after my first pit stop, but with each and every step thereafter, they began to feel a bit more intense. Around mile nine, I was really feeling the pain. I told Noel I might have to stop again. She was totally fine with that. Then I said, "Let's just take a little walk break until these cramps calm down or I can pass some gas and then I'll be good to go."

So we did. The less impact there was, the less pain I felt, so after a bit I suggested we run again. This continued for the next few miles, but eventually the walk breaks didn't help. The cramps were coming harder and faster, the pain was increasingly worse. They were ever present and wouldn't subside. Noel continued chatting about the scenery. We walked up and down the hills. I honestly don't remember much of the surroundings at that point. My mind was so focused on how much longer we had, nothing else registered. I was just trying to tune out the pain. I kept putting one foot in front of the other and telling myself, as I watched the mile markers pass by, I only have three more miles, I only have two more miles. I had one goal and that was to finish.

I held it in. I barely said a word those last two miles. I was in survival mode. This feeling was unlike any other I had experienced before, and I cringe to this day just thinking about it. I was so uncomfortable and about to explode as I crossed the finish line. I ran under the big FINISH banner and over the chip pad that recorded my time. As the volunteers pulled off my chip and hung a medal around my neck, I was doing my little bathroom dance. Squirmy and uncomfortable, I navigated through the crowd. Another volunteer tried to hand me a glass of wine. *OMG—No!* I broke free and B-lined to the bathroom. "I'll find you afterward," I yelled to Noel and kept running. I didn't look back.

I had to navigate my way through the vast park of porta-potties to look for the real deal because this business was too serious to take to a temporary facility (plus I would have likely fallen in since my quads just weren't strong enough to hold me up). I continued to run toward the ladies' restroom, while everyone around me was walking around, celebrating and exploring the vendor and winery kiosks that were set up in the finishers' village. I finally reached my concrete castle, and it was filled with multiple stalls. As if truly living a fairy tale, I couldn't wait to sit on my throne! Luckily the line wasn't too long. When I should have been focused on the enjoyment, accomplishment, and triumph of completing a half marathon, only pain consumed my thoughts. I pinched myself hard to divert my attention to an area of pain not emanating from inside my stomach. I kept crossing my legs as I stood in line, squeezing my butt cheeks together as I inched my way to the front.

I think I was in that stall for twenty minutes, maybe closer to thirty. I was thankful I was in California, at a race where I knew no one. Thankfully, I would never see these people again. I knew when I emerged from the stall, there would be no hiding my face. I had created the stall of shame. I just sat there, in so much pain. I couldn't get up. I folded myself in half on the toilet, bent over with cramps. When I started to sit upright, the cramps returned so I folded myself in half again. I was 100 percent depleted. Completely on empty. I'm sure I was dehydrated. I had nothing inside of me.

Making my way outside, I was dazed and confused, barely registering that I'd just completed a half marathon. I couldn't drink, not even water. I couldn't eat. I felt horrible. All around me people strolled from table to table sampling various wines, clinking their glasses. Music played in the background. Everyone was celebrating.

I returned to the finishers' expo to find Mark and Noel talking and enjoying themselves, ready to greet me with open arms. Mark was glad to see me. He had congratulated me as I crossed the finish line, but he obviously couldn't get past the barricades. He gave me a big hug and a kiss. I followed them as they walked along, checking out the various vendors. They kept asking me if I wanted anything. I told them that my stomach wasn't feeling well and left it at that. Noel left to meet her husband, Ted. She knew I was hurting and that I had struggled the last few miles. I don't think she realized the severity of my struggle. This race had felt much different than any of our other running adventures. Mark probably thought I was just tired. I knew better, though. I'd hit a turning point. I'd pushed myself too far, and my body was paying me back. The finish line I'd just crossed was likely to be one of my last, and the feelings I usually experienced after completing a race weren't present. No adrenaline rush, no elation, no pride. Instead, I felt despair and humility. I understood that my body was telling me I was finished and, this time, my mind had nowhere to run.

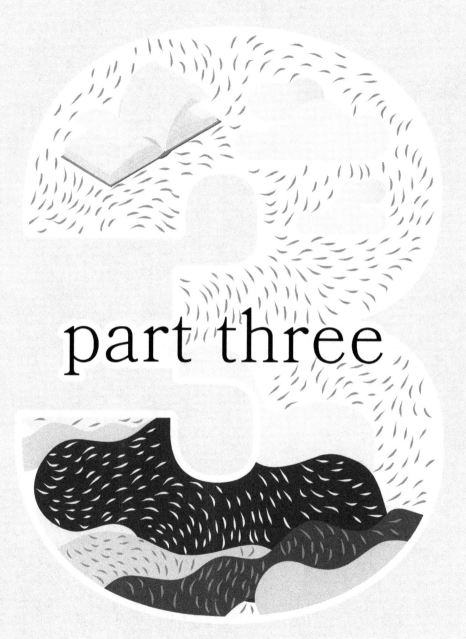

part three

part three

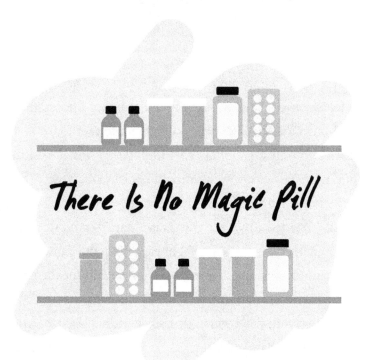

There Is No Magic Pill

ALMOST THIRTEEN MONTHS after my surgery in March of 2010, Mark and I took the vacation we'd planned before my Universal Intervention. Instead of going to a resort in California to lie by the pool drinking fruity drinks, we decided to head to Utah and check out Red Mountain Resort and Spa, where the vibe was a little more rustic and outdoorsy.

We hiked in the dessert, biked around town, practiced yoga, ate clean cuisine, and indulged in a spa treatment or two. But the most fascinating part of the trip wasn't the great outdoors as I had imagined it would be. The resort offered several possibilities for "personal discovery" as they called it. We could meet with energy healers, Tarot card readers, an iridologist, intuitives, tea leaf readers . . . I was so intrigued that I wanted to meet with them all, though Mark preferred sticking to the basics: attending yoga classes, stretch class, or swimming laps in the pool. I chose two, the Tarot card reader and the tea leaf lady. The women were lovely, positive, and provided me with what seemed like good insight and practical information at the time, although the specifics are now difficult to recall.

Then I got curious about the iridologist. Prior to visiting Red Mountain, I'd never heard of an iridologist. But when I read the description of what he offered, the voice deep within me started yelling again; I needed to go see this man. Mark was not overly positive about this, especially since I'd already seen the Tarot reader and the tea leaf lady. He questioned whether I really needed to make an appointment with a third practitioner. I researched a little more about iridology and determined that since iridologists look into your iris and tell you what's going on inside your body, it would give me another perspective on my digestive distress. I sensed a strong hunch that it would be helpful. So, on the last full day, I headed over to his office.

When I walked into the room, I was greeted by a man in his thirties with a calm demeanor. He looked me straight in the eye as he greeted me and asked me to sit down on the couch across from him and tell him a little bit about why I was there. I didn't want to divulge too much information. I wanted to test him a bit, to see if he could impress me with his abilities. I alluded to the fact that I'd had a major surgery within the last year, saying only that it had been a life-threatening situation, an emergency procedure, and that I was thankful the issue had been caught in time. I was still "sort of" getting back my health. I told him I was very active, a runner, former triathlete, and that I taught fitness classes. I also told him I was really dialed into my food. When I finally stopped talking, he quietly leaned forward and asked, "Do you have any digestive issues?"

Holy shit! Seriously? He'd just jumped about ten points in my credibility book. "Um, yes," I said, "quite a few." That began a long discussion about my gut. I spoke more specifically about the surgery, and after about fifteen minutes, he asked if I'd had my ileocecal valve removed, replaced, or severed and reattached.

"My what?" I knew I'd heard a similar term, ileoscopy, when the hospital staff referred to my surgery. I was pretty sure the doctor told me ten or maybe twenty times what he'd actually done during the procedure. But I was so doped up on pain meds during those days following the surgery, he might as well have told me he'd just delivered a unicorn because my reaction would have been the same: "Thanks so much, doc, for getting it out. I don't quite get all that you're saying right now, but I know I'm not in excruciating pain anymore. I just have a very large dressing on my mid-section that I'm not supposed to touch."

Since I wasn't sure, I told the iridologist that I didn't know. He proceeded to explain the importance of this valve in digestion and suggested I find out the answer as soon as I returned to Austin. This could be the reason I was still experiencing such gastric distress more than a year after surgery.

I didn't have to wait until I got back to Austin to investigate. I was on it! I went straight back to my room, googled the valve, its properties, and its importance. I discovered that without this valve, it's much more difficult for food to pass through the digestive tract because the valve acts as a sphincter. Kind of like a vacuum cleaner for your colon. It pulls everything down and helps to keep things moving. When the valve isn't operating or has been removed, food remains in the intestines and begins to rot, just like perishable food that's left out. This can create malabsorption problems. The toxins from malabsorbed food can then cause gas, bloating, belching, stomach pain (cramping), reflux, and several other symptoms. Thanks so much, Dr. Google!

I'm *such* a patient person that the next day, I awoke and even before brushing my teeth, I called the doctor's office to speak to someone who could tell me about my valve. "Just pull my chart and tell me what it says," I told the receptionist. "Did I or did I not have the ileocecal valve removed?" I totally thought she could look it up and tell me right then and there. But nope, not gonna happen! She said I'd need to address specific questions about the procedure with my surgeon, so I would have to make an appointment to see him. With much disgust and disappointment, I said, "Ugh, fine," and scheduled to meet with him the week following the trip. Then off I went to investigate my lost valve. Where was it? What had the surgeon done with it? If it was there, then why wasn't it working?

When I got to his office, I explained that even after fourteen months, I was still having the same, or possibly worse, issues with my digestion. The surgery hadn't seemed to remedy any of it. Then without hesitation, I asked, "Did you remove my ileocecal valve?" He told me he had, in fact, removed it and assured me this was not the reason I was still having problems digesting most foods. This was not why my stomach often became distended, nor why I produced so much gas and couldn't gain any weight.

"I take the valves out in all my colon cancer patients, the bad appendectomies I correct, and all my similar surgeries. That's not your problem."

And that was that. The moment he said, "That's not your problem," a lightbulb went on inside my head. Of course he didn't have any suggestions as to what my problem might be. A wave of strong emotion flooded me. I was grateful he'd saved my life but fuming that he'd lumped me and my surgery in with the mean of all past surgeries he'd performed. To me, his response sounded like an assumption: If no one else had issues with the removal of the valve, then there was no way it could be causing me problems. There was no individualized approach here. I knew there was something more to this puzzle and the removal of the valve seemed to be a huge piece.

From that day forward, I viewed allopathic medicine in a totally different light. I had no other choice but to figure this shit out for myself. I was energized by the information I'd received from the iridologist and the surgeon. It catapulted me to put on my sleuthing hat and take out my magnifying glass to begin to uncover, for myself, the real reason behind my digestive issues.

Over the next several months, I met with just about every holistic practitioner I could find who focused on the gut. Some in person, some over the phone. I sought out the best of the best: Gerard Mullin, Daniel Kalish, Chris Kresser. Those who had written books on the gut, those who were studying the gut-brain connection, those who educated me with their podcasts about gut dysbiosis (microbial imbalance). These were the practitioners my gut guided me to connect with. The functional medicine practitioners, gastroenterologists, the holistic doctors of osteopathic medicine (DOs) with practices focusing on the gut. I should have been keeping score—a hit, a strike, or a home run. Most were hits, gathering little nuggets of valuable information. I definitely struck out a few times, too, but I was constantly wishing and hoping for a home run. Then there were the spiritual healers, acupuncturists, and kinesiologists who appealed to me and were probably helping me more mentally than physically. I saw anyone and everyone I could find who might help me put together this massive puzzle. Sometimes I collected a piece or part of a piece, though most of the time I approached the situation full of hope but came out the other side devoid of any new earth-shattering information.

I made a phone call to a doctor in New York who I'd heard lecture on the gut. From describing my symptoms and from reading her a few markers from various labs I'd completed, she told me I wasn't absorbing any nutrients and that the supplements I was buying by the bagful were going in one end and out the other. I was literally peeing my money down the toilet, plain and simple.

A kinesiologist I'd been seeing referred me to an acupuncturist who dealt exclusively with patients experiencing gut issues. It didn't take me very long to look him up and make an appointment. I had a sneaking suspicion he'd be able to find something the others hadn't. I felt a little guilty "cheating" on Rosa, seeing another acupuncturist, but nothing could stop me. If he could shed any light on my shit, I had to know.

The day of my appointment, I was sitting in the exam room, when this goofy-looking, absent-minded, professor-like man entered the room. Once again, I told him about the issues I was having with my gut. At this point, a tape recorder would have been handy so I could just press play every time I saw a new practitioner. After listening to me, he treated me with needles, though he was convinced that parasites were strongly contributing to my poop problems. He said I would need something more than needles to banish the bugs. I was sure he was on to something. But things just got weirder from there. He began to explain that he worked very closely with a naturopath in Nigeria who used a powerful microscope to test for particular parasites and produced tinctures to eliminate them. While this should have probably raised a red flag, my naïveté and desire to destroy these devils was too strong to let any warning signals through. He could identify the different strains of parasites and once he knew exactly which parasites were partying in my gut, he'd dispense a tincture to rid me of them. Previous lab tests had confirmed the "probability" of parasites, though they did not test for the specific species.

I agreed to go ahead with the testing. The results confirmed his initial suspicions. "You have a number of parasites," he told me. Some were worms, others had scientific names I can't recall, and I also had the king of all parasites, Giardia. He began to explain the treatment protocol, and I wasn't sure if he was being serious or not. The Nigerian doctor would create tinctures for me to take based specifically on my lab results. It would take a couple weeks for him to concoct the individualized mixtures, after which they would be shipped to Austin. I was more than hopeful. *This is all beginning to make sense*, I thought. I excitedly told Mark about the new developments and patiently awaited the arrival of my package.

When I went to the office to pick up the tinctures, the accupuncturist handed me a bag containing six amber bottles filled with liquid. Each bottle had a strip of masking tape across the front. In black magic marker the letter A was written on three bottles and the letter B written on the others. I was to drink a half cup of each in the mornings and a half cup of each in the evenings, prior to any water or food. I had to finish both bottles completely. In the beginning, I might have symptoms like diarrhea or gas, but that was just the elimination of the critters from my body. "Okay," I said, bag of tinctures in hand, and happily off I went.

I got home and placed the bottles on my bathroom counter, ready to start the next morning. When I got up, I opened bottle A and almost passed out. It stunk to high heaven! I quickly screwed the lid on and held the bottle up to the light. Little flakes that looked like decomposed leaves and dead amoebas were floating around in the liquid. Trying not to think too much about the contents, I opened the bottle again, measured the dosage, and poured it into the cup sitting on the counter.

I picked up the cup. *Seriously, I'm supposed to drink this?* It smelled like a cross between rat urine and stale beer that had been fermenting for weeks. The closer the cup came to my nose, the more I felt like barfing. So, like any teenager about to take a shot of Jägermeister, I pinched my nose closed with one hand and threw the liquid down my throat with the other. Chaser, please! I grabbed a glass of water to remove the taste from my tongue as fast as I could. Then it was on to bottle B. I had eighteen more doses of this stuff, but who was counting? This was the potion with the motion to remove the gut bugs and get me back on track. I just knew it.

Two weeks later, back in the acupuncturist's office, we retested for the parasites. The results came back positive—the guys were still there! The doc explained that in my case, especially with the number of bugs I tested positive for, and particularly with the presence of Giardia, which is the most difficult to get rid of, I might have to repeat the protocol. *What?!?!?* He hadn't mentioned a second round before, but since I was clinging to all hope, I decided it made sense, kind of. So I agreed to do the whole damn thing again! I felt nauseated just thinking about it.

I went back to his office for a third test. Waiting for the results was painstakingly challenging. I didn't feel much different than I had after the first protocol, but I wanted to believe this round had done the trick. I sent all good vibes to the Universe while awaiting the results. The day of my appointment, I sat in his treatment room, biting my nails with nervous anxiety. When the door opened, the doc entered with his awkward stagger and a perplexed expression on his face. I watched as he flipped through my chart, squinting his eyes through his thick framed glasses. "Well," he mumbled, "it looks like we got rid of a few of the critters, though that Giardia, it's still holdin' on."

WTF? Seriously, dude! This was supposed to be it. No más!

"Are you and your husband active sexually?" he asked.

My stomach filled with dread. Things were getting stranger by the minute. He looked weird, had weird mannerisms, and was now asking weird questions. Creepy!

"You know parasites can be transmitted back and forth from person to person during intercourse. I suggest your husband go through a treatment as well."

That is SO not going to happen!

Throughout both treatments, my husband had constantly questioned my actions. "You're so careful about each and every little thing you put into your body. I can't believe you're drinking some strange concoction from an unlabeled bottle created by a so-called doctor that was supposedly flown in from another country. You have *no* idea what's in that and it smells G-d awful. Do you really think this is going to help?!?" He'd also left the room every time I'd opened the bottle to drink the stuff. That's how nasty it smelled.

"Do you think your husband would consider taking a round of the treatment?" the acupuncturist asked. "That way, we could rule him out as the cause. The parasite might not bother him, but with your compromised gut, it's taking a toll on you. I think it would be a good idea if you talked to him about it."

Half my brain was telling me how ridiculous this all sounded. *Am I seriously that gullible?* The other half of my brain was in that don't-give-up-when-you're-so-close-to-the-finish-line mode. This could be the determining factor. Don't give up hope after you've come this far! So later that evening, while Mark and I were cleaning up after dinner, I told him that the tincture was working, although the Giardia was still present. I could tell he'd heard about enough of my nonsense from an unnamed naturopath in Nigeria. His body language (arms crossed, leaning back) and energy exuded an air of disgust, frustration, and displeasure when I brought up the subject. I could tell this was not going to go well, but I was *not* going to give up! I was *sooo* close to the finish line. One more round for each of us and I would be in the clear. I was clinging to all hope.

"So, the guy said that because we're sexually active, we could be passing the parasites back and forth to one another. He wants us both to go through the protocol together to rule that out as a means of transmission. You in?!?!?"

Silence.

"I really think it's going to work," I rushed on. "I'll never know if we don't try. Could you? Would you? Please?"

"Let me think about it," he said.

With a hope and a prayer, I waited. A day or two later, I followed up with Mark. I'm certain I had thrown some comments, reminders, and inquiries out there in the interim, but this time I asked him directly. "Well?"

"Okay," he sighed, "I'll do it. But I'm not very pleased about it at all."

"Oh my G-d! Thank you so much!" I hugged him and told him I knew it was really gross, but if I could do this *three* times, he could handle it once.

If that doesn't show true love, I'm not really sure what does. He's not one to send flowers, but when it comes to drinking unlabeled, imported rat piss, he's definitely my man!

Mark never had to drink the stuff. While I waited for the third round of liquids to arrive, I wavered between hope and despair, but mainly despair. I began to feel dejected, gloomy, and incredibly frustrated. The promise this peculiar practitioner held for me began to decay like the smell of the putrefied tincture. I had to face it, if two rounds hadn't helped, a third wouldn't either. I'd had it. And when the package arrived, I shoved it to the back of a cabinet, later pouring it down the drain. I wasn't absorbing nutrients. I wasn't gaining weight. My digestion was still a mess. Months and even years after the surgery, nothing had changed. I couldn't run. I mean I ran, but it felt awful. I was getting increasingly depressed about the fact that nobody could really help me feel better. These practitioners just kept putting me on schedules and treatments that hadn't worked, so I stopped following them. They had been prescribing a shit ton of supplements that cost a crapload of money, which I was literally pissing away. I kept thinking, *I shouldn't be this exhausted. I shouldn't have this much bloating, gas, and bowel elimination. I shouldn't feel like crap constantly. Why can't anyone freaking figure me out?*

At this point, I had seen every Eastern and Western practitioner in Austin that I knew existed. I decided to consult a highly touted gastroenterologist, Gerard Mullin, at Johns Hopkins in Baltimore, whom Rosa had heard speak at a conference. I flew up with Mark for a long weekend. After a battery of tests, including bloodwork, a breath test to detect Small Intestinal Bacterial Overgrowth (SIBO), and a full endoscopy, he shed more light on why, in fact, my body was in its current state of affairs. The results from the endoscopy showed that the villi, the little hair-like protrusions that line the interior of the colon, were so withered that instead of the lining of my small intestine looking like velvet, it had the appearance of a stained concrete floor. The villi help the absorption of food by secreting enzymes that help breakdown the nutrients in food. When they become damaged, symptoms like diarrhea, weight loss, and anemia may occur.

Well, that was an *A-ha!* moment for sure! The enzymes weren't being produced to help break down the food and the remains of the food in my gut were causing the symptoms. Since the nutrients weren't being absorbed because the food I ate was basically sliding right out, I wasn't gaining any weight. Dr. Mullin suggested I take digestive enzymes with every meal to help me break down and more easily absorb my food. I began this protocol immediately though, sadly, I experienced little improvement.

I was at my wit's end, and Mark had had enough of my seeing all these woo-woo doctors. I'd cleaned out an entire shelf in our pantry to house all the supplements I was taking, which, we both knew, were doing nothing for me. He'd been asking around about other doctors from friends in the medical field. Steve, the friend he'd called when I was in the hospital, suggested someone. One afternoon, after the kids had retreated to their rooms and we were discussing the week ahead, Mark told me about her and asked that I go see her.

"No," I said. "Why should I go? No." I didn't know a thing about her.

He told me she was an internist and that he'd already made an appointment for both of us to go. He insisted I see her. "We've spent so much money on these practitioners," he said, "and you're still not better. The least you can do is go see this woman who comes highly recommended by someone in the field."

I didn't say a word. I was just so sick of being poked and prodded and not making any forward progress.

"We have an appointment next Tuesday at 2:00 p.m. I'll come home early from work and we can go together." He was putting his foot down, which rarely happens. He wasn't going to back down and this made me even more upset.

Furious, I grabbed my keys to run a few errands. I ran by People's Pharmacy to pick up a prescription. People's is a highly respected compound pharmacy. They prepare customized medications based on the practitioner's prescription. They also sell pharmaceutical-grade supplements, grass-fed beef, and serve sand-

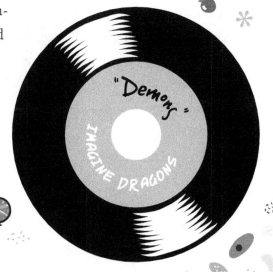

wiches, soups, and salads. I completely forgot they closed at 5:00 that day, so by the time I got there, they were about to lock up. Beth, a naturopath I'd met in the restorative yoga class I was taking when I had my surgery, saw me as I was headed back towards the pharmacy.

"How are you feeling?" she asked.

The yoga class where we'd met had been small and intimate, for women only. We'd shared quite a bit about ourselves in the short time we were together. Beth was soft-spoken, smart, and seemed like someone who was always there to lend a helping hand. She had a small frame, but her eyes were big and full of compassion.

I looked at her, at the shelves of supplements behind her. "I'm feeling about the same. I'm freaking frustrated."

"Why?" she asked.

"There's nobody who can help me," I said. Everyone who inquired about my health had been providing advice, recommending doctors. I would just tell them flat out that I'd been to every good holistic practitioner in Austin, I'd done my due diligence, and there was no one in this city competent enough to take on my complex issues. I figured I'd have to continue looking beyond Austin for specialists I felt comfortable seeing. I had begun the inquiry process, and had already filled out paperwork to see the well-known functional medical doc, Mark Hyman in Lenox, Massachusetts, although he had a six-month waiting list at the time.

Beth turned and walked toward her desk. "I've got a recommendation for you," she said over her shoulder.

I was about to wring her neck. That's the last thing I wanted to hear. "Somebody in Austin?" I mentally rolled my eyes.

146

She said, "Yeah," and I told her to forget it. I'd seen them all. Beth pulled a card out of her drawer and handed it to me anyway. The card said Mark Dickey, MD, Holistic Family Medicine. "This guy's really good," she said. "He practices a combination of Eastern and Western medicine. You might want to call him."

"Thanks," I muttered as I took the card and quickly walked toward the cashier. The guy behind the counter was already turning out the lights. I paid for the prescription, walked out the door, got into my car, put my key in the ignition, and looked down into my open purse for the business card Beth had handed me. I spotted the bag with the prescription in it, but no card. I felt a swirl of panic. An impulse drew me back into the store. When Beth first handed me the card, I was like, *Whatever, another practitioner* . . . But suddenly, I had to find it. I knew I had to have it. I dug through my purse. Still no card. I looked between the seats. No card. I checked the floor. *Where is that friggin' card?* I got out of my car, ran back to the pharmacy, and yanked on the door. It was locked. The lights were off. I started banging on the thick glass.

One of the staff was at the register, counting his drawer, and he looked at me, as though to say, "Hellooo, lady. We're closed."

I didn't care. I had to have that card. I stuck my head up against the glass and tented my hands above my eyes. I can only imagine what my face looked like to this guy, smashed against the glass, semi-hysterical. I saw the card lying on the counter. I started pointing, tapping my finger against the glass. "I know you're closed," I yelled. "I left something on the counter." I had no idea if he had a clue what I was saying. He finally opened the door but blocked the entrance.

"That card, on the counter," I said, "can you please get it for me? Beth gave it to me and I left it there." He turned around, got the card, and handed it to me. I thanked him profusely, ran back to the car, grabbed my cell phone and immediately dialed Dr. Dickey's number. It was late Sunday afternoon, so I left a message.

The next morning, I was in my bedroom when I got a phone call from Dr. Dickey's wife, Hazel, who happened to run the office. I sat on my bed, and we proceeded to talk for an hour. We'd had many similar issues, GI problems, for which we'd both had emergency surgery. I was dumbfounded. I felt the Universe had just stepped in to help me out. There was a reason I got that card, a reason I was speaking with this woman now instead of the doctor, a reason we'd had a very similar experience. Everything seemed preordained. Without hesitation, I made an appointment for the following week.

I felt my spirits lift almost instantly. This could be the answer. When Mark came home and asked me about my day, I told him about the conversation.

"I talked with a woman whose husband is a holistic practitioner and—"

"No." He interrupted me before I could finish, his brow furrowed and a look of disgust on his face.

"No? No, what?" I asked. *You cannot bring me down right now, dude. I'm flying high!* I could feel my blood pressure starting to rise. "No. You're seeing Dr. Adams. We have an appointment tomorrow."

We? "You know I don't want to go. It's the last thing I want to do. She's not going to be able to help me."

"She can help," Mark said. "She and I have discussed what's going on with you."

"You talked to her about me? Why would you do that?"

"Ellen, we're at our wits' end. We're going."

I kept saying I didn't want to go and he kept insisting we were. We had a huge fight and didn't speak two words to each other the rest of the evening. The next day, I caved, only to appease him, but I wasn't happy about it. I drove with Mark to the appointment in silence. I'm sure he could see the steam emitting from my ears. The nurse took me to the back, weighed me, measured my height, took my blood pressure—all the standard Western protocol, then Mark and I waited for the doctor in one of her examination rooms. We sat and listened to the hum of the fluorescent lights above us, neither saying a word. The doctor finally entered the room and shook my hand, looked me over, and reviewed the information I had filled out on my intake form.

She sat quietly in her white coat, flipping through pages and pages of lab results from recent tests I'd brought with me. We went through a bit of Q & A about symptoms and how I'd been feeling, but I could tell she'd already formed an opinion of the situation before I had even arrived. After a little more small talk, she suggested I check into a treatment facility for anorexia.

"Say *what*?" My mouth dropped open, a look of disgust filled my face. I was completely humiliated and repulsed. Tears welled in my eyes.

"How long would you be comfortable being away from your family?" she asked me.

"What?! Are you being completely serious?" I had a feeling I was living a bad dream.

"There are a lot of great places I can guide you to that can help you. We can get you back on track. We can get some weight on you. You're way too thin and your restrictive eating behavior is driving all your issues. You'll feel better. Your depression will subside. Everything will start coming together."

I just stared at her. I had nothing to say. Well, I did, though it wouldn't have been appropriate in this situation. "Your husband is very worried about you." She exchanged a look with Mark. "He's here to support you. He's willing to let you go for any amount of time it takes." She paused, waiting for my response.

I was pissed that *she* was telling *me* what *my* husband felt. I loathed that they'd talked about me. "I am *not* leaving my family for three days, three weeks, or three months for treatment of something I don't have."

She looked a bit smug. "Yes," she said.

Mark was quiet during most of the discussion, but he confirmed that there were food issues—eating alone, avoiding certain foods, and continuing to remove trigger foods from my diet. He, too, thought there was an underlying eating disorder driving all the problems I was having. He wanted something that would help me feel better, to get me to return to my former weight and my cheery ol' self.

"There are a lot of different issues here and the staff at the facility can help to get you back on track with your digestion and get you on a plan so that you can be eating . . ." Blah, blah, blah. I heard her but refused to listen.

Oh, my G-d. The entire visit went on like that. I'd speak up. She'd wave away my feelings as textbook responses and continue on her mission of getting me into treatment. I felt defensive and self-protective the entire time, growing more furious after I left. I was deeply upset and could barely speak to Mark on the drive home. I was so angry with him for taking me there. I was so caught up in my own emotions that any ability to see beyond them was obscured.

Later that week, I went to see my energy healer, Nancy. She was more like a therapist to me. I told her about the visit to Dr. Adams and Mark's reaction to my decision to make an appointment with Dr. Dickey.

"Mark loves you and hopes that going through treatment will improve your condition," she said, "and you have a huge support system. What about that is making you feel bad?"

I had no idea. "I don't know. My head is so confused, and I have no idea what's really going on in my body. I don't know if I have an eating disorder or if my body is a mess because of digestive issues. I just don't know." I knew I had issues with food, but I also knew I wasn't battling anorexia. I'd never considered one of these treatment facilities because my food limitations stemmed from the digestive discomfort I experienced after eating.

After seeing Nancy, I felt more confused than ever. Was everyone else right and I just couldn't see what was going on with me? Was I in denial? The more I thought about my situation, the more I began to believe that I actually did have a disorder that was worthy of treatment, an isolated, take-me-out-of-my-environment treatment for an intense, yet transformational approach to healing. Maybe my food restrictions and exercise addiction really required a "retreat."

One night, after the kids and Mark were in bed, I took my iPad, sat at the kitchen island, and started researching every single treatment facility in the United States. With filters, of course. It had to be green. They had to serve organic food. They had to offer yoga and meditation. I wasn't going to an institutional facility with four white walls and doctors in white coats. Nothing sterile. Something in nature. I wanted to go to a place where I would be among similar-minded people. Those who shared the same values as I did, and possibly the same issues.

After hours of googling, I finally stopped about 1:00 a.m. I'd found a couple of places that looked somewhat appealing. When I went to see Nancy again, I reported my findings, which she thought were great options. But after I left her office, and the more I really thought about going, the more I realized how wrong a treatment facility felt. *What the hell am I thinking?* I asked myself. *This is not okay. I'm not going. Am I crazy? I am NOT uprooting myself from my family for three months!* An eating disorder was not the major issue. But I wasn't sure what the major issue was. I couldn't wrap my head around the fact that I felt so terrible and nobody could heal me. I was going to give it one last shot with Dr. Dickey.

The night before my appointment with Dr. Dickey, Mark and I were lying in bed when he asked me what I was doing the next day.

"I have that appointment with Dr. Dickey," I said.

"You're still planning on seeing him? Really?" he asked, clearly exasperated.

"I went to the doctor you wanted me to see. Now you can come with me to the doctor I want to see," I said.

"No. I'm not going," he said. "We've talked about this repeatedly. You're not going. Don't even think about it."

I didn't say a word. I was going. No one could stop me. I turned over and went to sleep.

The next morning, I'd just taken a shower and was getting ready to go to the appointment, when Mark entered the bathroom and asked, once again, about my plans for the day.

"You know good and well what I'm doing today. I'm going to this appointment."

He asked me what time it was scheduled.

"I told you. It's at 9:30 this morning." I walked out of the bathroom, got the kids' stuff together, and took them to school. I had about an hour before the appointment so I came back home to get my paperwork together. I stuffed files, lab work, test results, a notebook, and my intake form into a canvas bag. This was the last resort. *Make it or break it,* I thought. I had a good feeling about him after talking to his wife on the phone and I was holding on to that supposition with a hope and a prayer.

As I pulled up to his office, a small little house close to the university, I saw Mark's car in the parking lot. That's interesting, I thought. When I opened the door to the house and entered the waiting room, Hazel came out from behind the desk and gave me a hug. It was like we were old friends who hadn't seen each other in a while, or, in reality, ever. Mark was in the waiting room, too. He was sitting in a chair leafing through a magazine, looking a little uncomfortable. I looked at him and tried to hide the smirk on my face.

Shortly after, Dr. Dickey came to greet us. He was about our age, maybe a few years older. Grey hair and a beard. He was wearing jeans, a short-sleeve button-down, and Birks. "Come on back," he said after shaking both of our hands.

We walked back into what had probably been the master bedroom of the old house.

"Have a seat." He gestured toward the two leather chairs, then sat behind his big wooden desk, facing us. It was a very homey office—wood floors, leather chairs, oriental rug, and two large bookshelves filled top to bottom with health books, many of which I had in my personal library—Nourishing Traditions, Grain Brain, The China Study, The Food Revolution, Healing with Whole Foods. I already felt at ease.

"Well," he said, leaning forward, "what can I do you for? Hazel mentioned that you had some gut issues and have also had an ileoscopy. When was that?"

I talked through my entire health history, my surgery, my current state of affairs, including all the holistic practitioners I'd seen and consulted with, and discussed the multitude of supplements I had taken or was currently taking. I told him about the woo-woo acupuncturist who had tested me for parasites and prescribed an unknown mixture of substances imported from another practitioner in Nigeria. Dr. Dickey just nodded as I spoke. He listened and interspersed a few questions in my long dissertation when I paused for a breath. I felt like he needed to know *everything*. And I told him everything, including my frustrations. As I talked, it seemed as though he understood me. I felt a connection to him that I hadn't felt with any other doctor. He seemed real. He wanted to learn about me. His questions were specific to my symptoms, my struggles, my protocol. I felt an enormous sense of relief. I looked at Mark periodically as I spoke. He too seemed comfortable with Dickey's comments. I laughed a little, feeling such a sense of hope that my eyes filled with tears. I just kept thinking, *He gets it. He understands. Okay. Finally!!!*

He looked at me and said, "So you had major surgery because your colon was tied in a knot. You lost your ileocecal valve. You have Giardia among several other parasites . . . You've basically been shooting BB guns at these issues for so long, it's time to pull out the M16s."

That didn't sound good. "What do you mean?"

"You can do acupuncture. You can drink tinctures. You can take Chinese herbs, supplements, oils . . . that's all great, but when you have several different issues all occurring in the system concurrently, you've got to make a plan, prioritize. My suggestion would be to hit these parasites hard with some really serious antibiotics and then you'll start to feel better."

At one time, I would have fought against antibiotics, but at that point, I heard him loud and clear. There was a time and place for Western medicine and this was the time. My time. I had a freaking stomach full of bugs who were having a huge frat party and I needed to blow them out of my system. "Okay, fine," I said. "That all makes sense." I began see light at the end of the tunnel.

Mark checked his watch. "It's almost noon and I have a phone call back at the office."

What? You're kidding. We'd been in his office for over two hours? It felt like forty-five minutes. Seriously, what doctor gives you that kind of time and attention?

Mark stood up. "I'm going to have to excuse myself. It was great meeting you, doctor. Thank you so much for your insight. Ellen, I'll call you later." I could tell he was just as relieved as I was. It seemed as though we both felt Dr. Dickey had the knowledge and the ability to set me on the right path.

I ended up staying for a total of three hours. Dr. Dickey and I talked for another half hour about my specific plan. He gave me a prescription for two high-potency antibiotics that I would start taking the following week during the full moon. "Parasites are more active during the full moon cycles," he commented. I totally loved how he thought. We agreed to set up another appointment after I finished my course of medication. I let out a big sigh of relief as I left his office and prayed that I had correctly perceived Mark's positive feelings toward Dr. Dickey.

I was right. Mark thought the treatment made sense, too, and agreed with my decision to take the antibiotics to try and kill off the Giardia. It was a four-day protocol. I felt a shift both in my body and my brain after the course of drugs was complete. I started to gain a bit more clarity and perspective about myself and my choices. It was subtle, though enough that I began to alter my behavior. I listened to my body when it was yelling at me not to run. The constant bloat I carried in my belly lessened a bit. I became curious and, it seemed, more intuitive.

When I returned to Dickey's office, I told him I was starting to feel better, and he said, "Great!" then added, "I know you. I know you really well, your type, that is. And I know what's going to happen. Once you start to feel better, you are going to go back into your daily routine. Pushing harder, running longer. I'm not going to let you walk out of this office and return to your former pattern. It's not what your body needs right now. You have to allow the time and the space to let your body, your mind, and your gut heal. There are multiple issues you're dealing with. You need accountability so you're going to be accountable to me, do you understand? No more running. No more raw foods."

He looked stern, an expression I hadn't seen during our first meeting. He wasn't messing around. I felt both afraid and thankful. I needed boundaries and I knew it. I couldn't place them upon myself so this was literally *just* what the doctor ordered.

I nodded. "This is exactly what I need," I said. "I need somebody to hold me accountable." And once again, I felt understood. I felt hope. I saw light.

"I know you do, so I'm telling you that you'll follow a specific exercise protocol and you'll go to a nutritionist."

"Okay." I gulped.

Dr. Dickey recommended I work with a personal trainer and suggested Mark Herbert, who also rented a space in his building. "You've lost a lot of strength," he said, "a lot of muscle. You're very weak and thin. I want you to gain your strength back, but in a very smart and calculated manner. Do not run, do not run, do not run. You're not allowed to run. I'll introduce you to Mark on the way out. He's going to be watching you and he will be reporting back to me. Mark, the trainer, your nutritionist, you, and I—we're all going to be working together. As a team."

Mark the trainer was cool. In my first session, he started me off with basic form and function. I didn't break a sweat. I was kind of annoyed (or very annoyed) that I was paying good money for someone to tell me how to stand and how to squat as he placed a stick against my back for postural alignment, instructing me to open my thoracic spine. I think he could tell I was slightly irritated. I didn't say too much during that session. I just followed his commands. I probably asked a few times for more weight and more intensity, and he allowed it within reason. So I went back. During those initial sessions, we talked about training and created a bond, a mutual respect. I, too, was a personal trainer and we valued each other's knowledge and wisdom. He also was a science nerd who loved to geek out on nutrition and the gut, so our discussions were something I began to look forward to as well. As I continued to gain strength, he continued to challenge me and I stuck with him.

I had made an appointment to see the nutritionist Dickey suggested. I was doing my best to keep my thoughts neutral and open to someone telling me what to eat . . . once again. When we first met, she seemed to have an air about her, kind of like she knew everything. I dismissed it and kept telling myself to listen, to be open, and to learn. She handed me a spiral-bound notebook, the front half was like a workbook and the back was sort of like a cookbook, filled with the recipes she'd created and wanted me to cook and eat. While some seemed doable, others like Portobello burgers, rosemary lentil cakes, and coconut flour pancakes weren't as appealing. She wanted me to start filling out the workbook by journaling my food and my body's reaction to the food after cooking some of the recipes. We would meet again in a week.

This continued for a month or so until my next appointment with Dickey. I told him that Mark and I were working out weekly and that things were going well. "The nutritionist, on the other hand, not so much. I don't think our personalities align." I appreciated her information and what she was offering, but I had an intuitive feeling that she wasn't very knowledgeable when it came to my specific issues and their complexities. And, in addition, I really didn't like her attitude. I asked his permission to not go back, and he agreed.

Dr. Dickey continued to see an upward trend in my progress and commended me for my efforts. He invited me to listen to my body and fuel it with the foods I knew were healing, nourishing, and satiating. He continued to order labs and test for the parasites, which had not returned. The focus now was on rebuilding my gut after several years of being in a state of dysbiosis. On top of the parasite issues, other tests had confirmed candida and a large overgrowth of yeast, among other gut issues. He was very patient, as I was not, and continued to take time explaining the next steps in my healing protocol. Weeks and months passed. I was gaining weight and strength. The weight was coming back on slowly and steadily, just as he had planned. He knew me well and understood both the physical and mental components of the transition. Sometimes we have to step back, take a deep breath, and trust the not only the Universe, but those it sends to guide us and help us navigate our way.

I learned that the acceptance of my diagnoses, the trust I placed in others and in the process, the gratitude for finding a healing path, and being honest with myself and my issues created the prescription for the realization that there is no magic pill.

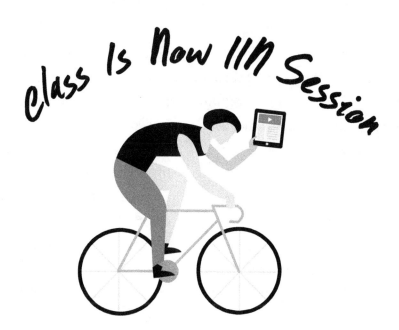

Class Is Now IIN Session

ONE OF MY FAVORITE PLACES in the world is Chautauqua Institution in New York state. Each summer, my family and I rent a condo there and spend two weeks attending lectures, the ballet, the opera, the symphony, and the theater. It's magical, I absolutely love it there. The recreation programs abound and include everything from tennis and sailing to canoeing and lawn bowling. Kids attend the oldest day camp in the nation, The Boys & Girls Club. Teens hang out at the Youth Activity Center (YAC). The YAC coordinates scavenger hunts, themed dances, overnight canoe trips, and best of all, Air Band competitions, where the kids dress up, take the stage as a famous band of their choice, and play air guitars. It's awesome.

The community is highly intellectual—a large percentage of attendees are professors, doctors, and scientists from all over the country. The Special Studies program offers classes in the culinary, visual, and theater arts; business and finance; computer; dance; health and fitness; and writing, just to name a few. Classes are taught by visiting lecturers, professors, and guests at Chautauqua who passionately share their professional knowledge with others. The people I meet there are some of the nicest and most welcoming I've ever known. There are concerts every Friday night at the Amp, including The Beach Boys, The Avett Brothers, Sheryl Crow, Jay Leno, and Aretha Franklin, to name a few. Each of the nine weeks has a theme around which the lectures are based: Invention, The Nature of Fear, Our Changing Relationship with Food, The Art of Play, American Identity, The Ethics of Dissent. I've heard amazing speakers: editors from *The New York Times*, Supreme Court justices, TV personalities, media moguls, authors, comics, scientists, anthropologists, explorers, religious figures. Each and every summer, my mind is sufficiently blown.

I describe Chautauqua as a Disney World for adults. There's a unicorn-like air circulating the grounds. It's where I came up with the name for my business, The Locavore Next Door, and where I wrote a large part of this book. There I can relax, restore, refresh, and recharge my system.

When I'm on the grounds, my connection to nature is heightened, beautiful flowers are blooming, storms are brewing, birds are chirping, the lake glistens as the sun sets over the horizon. I visit many local farms—harvesting garlic, picking blueberries, learning about growing mushrooms and making wine. There's a tremendous appreciation for locally grown food. I cook . . . a lot! I shop at several farmers markets in the area and creatively utilize the local bounty in my kitchen.

I practice yoga almost every morning, by myself, sometimes in the rec center, other times overlooking the lake, where I appreciate the cool breeze blowing above me and the dewy grass beneath my feet. I feel as though I'm making deposits into my chill account, which I deplete steadily throughout the year.

We all come and go as we please. There aren't many cars. People walk everywhere or ride their bikes. We leave doors unlocked, windows open. The kids are free to wander and hang out with friends. Adults typically go to the evening programs or gather together on someone's porch, nibbling on locally made cheese and sipping wine, picking up where they left off the year prior.

Our first trip to Chautauqua was in 2011, the summer before I started seeing Dr. Dickey, and about six months after I found out about the removal of my ileocecal valve. I was still feeling awful, was incredibly frustrated, and hoped that the time away would alleviate some of the stress I constantly carried with me. While we were there, I took a special studies class on the chakras. There were about eight to ten people in attendance. We introduced ourselves in the beginning of class and talked about why each of us chose the course. I briefly spoke about my surgery. I expressed the desire to tap into my own energy and open the channels flowing through my chakras. Both Kerry and Rosa often spoke about my blocked chakra energy, especially my root chakra (groundedness), my throat chakra (communication), and my heart chakra (love and connection). Nancy, my energy healer, also worked to open, balance, and repattern my chakra energy.

After class that day, a woman who had mentioned she was a health coach approached me as I was leaving. We started talking about nutrition, the gut, supplements, fermented foods, and functional medicine. I shared more about my surgery and my quest to improve my compromised digestion. I told her about all the practitioners I was seeing to help me manage these symptoms, though I was convinced there was much more to uncover, learn, and explore. She told me about an online health coaching certification she had received from the Institute for Integrative Nutrition (IIN). Bursting with enthusiasm, she spoke about the training and encouraged me to sign up. She thought the class would help me discover some of the answers I'd been searching for. "You would be the perfect candidate!" she said.

The Institute for Integrative Nutrition is a yearlong course. After completing forty modules and taking four exams, you become certified as a health coach. There are hundreds if not thousands of people who go through the program at once, all with different backgrounds, priorities, and aspirations. You have an automatic network of people with whom you can work, study, ask questions, and share experiences.

"This is so weird that you're mentioning this," I said. "I've had a brochure on my desk from IIN for about six months." When I first received the catalogue in the mail, I pored over the description of classes: some looked at the connection between our spiritual and emotional selves, others explored dietary theories, mindful eating, modified crops, vitamins, minerals and macronutrients, love as medicine, how to eliminate food sensitivities, issues of absorption and digestion, sugar addiction. *Oh, my gosh,* I thought. *I so want to do this!!!* I read through every word of their website. I had even called the office to find out the cost of the program. I noted some of the names of the impressive speakers who contributed to the program—Deepak Chopra, Andrew Weil, Geneen Roth, Walter Willett, Sally Fallon, Julia Ross, Bernie Seigel, David Katz, and Mark Hyman.

But I couldn't justify the price. Plus, I figured it would require between ten to twenty hours a week and I had no idea how to carve that kind of time out of my schedule. So instead of just tossing the catalogue in the recycling bin, I shoved it to the side of my desk, thinking, *Someday, I'm going to take this course*, though I had no idea how or when. The physical catalogue became a reminder of the emotional and energetic connection I felt to this class.

After thanking her for the heartfelt advice, I raced back to our condo. I was so excited. I was certain that the time was right. I could make this work. I *would* make this work. Her words were confirmation that all this valuable information could definitely impact the future of my health. I was smiling from the inside out, glowing with enthusiasm from our conversation. The minute I walked in the front door, I grabbed my phone, closed the door to the bedroom, and called IIN. I wrote down all the information in my notebook, from optional payment plans and possible start dates to enrollment numbers and anticipated time commitment per week. I was intrigued by the courses and teachers, fascinated by all I could learn. I wanted to gain more nutritional wisdom that would help me catapult my healing into a different zone. It would heal my stomach, and since the course was geared toward training health practitioners, maybe once I was healed, I could help others who had similar issues.

After I hung up the phone, I went into the living room, where Mark was working, and told him I wanted to commit to the course. I was a bit nervous to bring it up, especially since it carried a hefty price tag. I also knew I would get some slack about adding "one more thing" to my plate. Mark listened attentively as I debated my point, but he wasn't exactly overflowing with enthusiasm. When I finished he said, "Ellen, are you kidding me? It's a huge commitment. You're supposed to be slowing down. Plus, it's not cheap. What would you do with this certificate, anyway?"

I wasn't sure exactly what my intentions were other than to learn, absorb, and apply the knowledge to improve my personal health. I felt such a strong emotional magnetism to the course. I was pursuing all leads at that point, tugging on every string available to unravel the knot of whatever the hell was going on with me. I was determined, and not at all diplomatic. "I'm going to do this," I said, "I'll figure it out. I'll make time, and not at the expense of you and the kids. This is to help me heal. I'm at my breaking point. I know this course will lead me to answers that no one else can provide." The conversation had deflated my enthusiasm but hadn't completely busted my bubbly fervor. Exasperated, but not discouraged, I left the room. I returned to my computer, clicking through the IIN website, reading the testimonials, and regaining my excitement about taking the course.

When we returned to Austin, my first order of business—other than laundry, paying bills, and getting back into the normal routine—was to enroll in the next course, which began in September. I felt incredibly excited to start. I couldn't stop talking about it. After I registered, they sent a number of foundational classes to listen to prior to the start of the program. At the same time, those enrolled in the course began to connect via social media. The discussion threads were so incredibly long that one couldn't possibly keep up with all the responses, which came fast and furious, 24/7.

Once the course began, I received new modules every week. Each module contained lectures, assignments, videos, and exercises. After each set of ten modules, there was an exam. We were encouraged to join a study/support group, and I was lucky enough to find a small group of women in Austin who had started the program in September, the same time I had. We'd meet at coffee shops to discuss our progress, our assignments, how well we were (or weren't) practicing with our mock clients—friends, neighbors, and acquaintances who'd agree to let us try out what we were learning. Occasionally we would cook together, using the recipes and techniques we had received with the most recent lecture. We would also study together prior to the exams.

I wasn't always thrilled by the modules. Some modules focused on nutrition, some on mindfulness, breath, yoga, and grounding. In each module there was at least one lecture about how to start your health coaching practice, how to set up your website, how to practice with clients, attract clientele, and how to use social media to market and promote your business. I didn't find those mind-blowing. That's not where my interest lay. Then there were all the practicums—individual health coaching and group health coaching. They encouraged us to practice, practice, practice—but not, under any circumstances, on our family, spouse, or relatives because of the deep emotional connection we shared. There would be too much baggage to be objective. But when I tried practicing on some of my current personal training clients, it felt awkward. I kept thinking, *Wow, this isn't resonating with me. I don't think I want to become a health coach. That's not why I'm taking the course. It's not what I want to do. I just want to gather information.* I completed my assignments and listened to the modules in their entirety, though I mainly focused on the material that I believed could help me heal.

I studied in my workout studio. Before we had built the studio, I'd been training clients in the gym, and yearned for a space of my own to teach and train. We'd lived in our house for almost a year when we decided to convert the old carport at the back of the house to a workout studio. I designed it myself—from the layout to the music station to the bamboo wall where I attached bands and ropes to inlaid wall clips that provided different angles and degrees of resistance for my clients. The studio ended up more beautiful than I ever expected. It looked out over our pool and the vegetable garden. The doors were large sliding barn doors that I sometimes left open to let the outdoors in. It was the perfect size for both individual sessions and my small group classes. Occasionally, when I had overflow, I left the doors open and created stations for the clients to rotate through, some inside and some out. I loved that studio—my own private space, away from the doorbell and the dirty laundry. For three and a half years, from the time we built it until we moved, that was my favorite part of the house. During the year of my IIN class, I would retreat into my studio on Saturday mornings to listen to the weekly modules.

While I watched and listened to these modules, I rode my old triathlon bike that was hooked up to the CompuTrainer I had bought when I was training for triathlons. It's a computer program that communicates with the bike through wires attached to the bike stand. The CompuTrainer manipulates a device in the rear of the stand to provide more resistance when you're simulating a hill and releases tension when you're descending. Along with the scenery, the screen displays a little man on a bike, the pacer, whom you ride against. You are supposed to keep up with him or pass him, though I was no longer in training mode, so I didn't care how far ahead of me he was. I was only concerned with completing the entire profile and spending several hours on the bike.

The speakers who discussed food and exercise addiction, depression, recovery, and the ways they learned to ground themselves, meditate, and balance were some of my favorites. I was enthralled with all the different narratives—people with different backgrounds and experiences, some well-known speakers and authors, talking about how nutrition, yoga, and mindfulness changed their lives. They discussed how they overcame personal issues they had remained silent about for so long. If a lecture really resonated with me, I would listen to it three or four times on my iPod when I walked the dog, folded laundry, ran errands, or picked up kids. Sometimes I would be listening to the speakers recount the healing benefits of slowing down, sitting quietly, meditating, listening to their bodies—and I'd just cry.

I had heard this advice for years and knew deep down that it was true—stop running, stop moving constantly, quit expending so much energy and getting involved in so many activities. Slow down. Breathe. Take it easy. As I rode, my mind yammered: *This makes so much sense! Put your head in the game, Ellen! The food and nutrition piece are a large component but if your lifestyle and mindset remain in constant motion, you may not ever get better.* I thought, as I sped along in a race by myself: *There's a reason I'm listening to this.*

It's not that I didn't get the irony of spinning my wheels for hours every Saturday while listening to lectures about slowing down, tuning in, finding balance. But what was my alternative? To sit on a chair in front of my computer and watch the speaker lecturing at the podium? Um, not gonna happen. No way. Not even at my most vulnerable point, with heightened awareness about the disorder I possessed, could I picture being that person. And I needed my workout. So the way I saw it, I was killing two birds with one stone. And somehow, moving my body while I watched and listened felt like a moving meditation. Feeling the circular pedal strokes over and over and over again, identifying with the speakers' histories as I cried, I began to truly integrate this message about listening to my body, which is one of the reasons, I think, aside from being at my wit's end, I was so ready to listen to Dr. Dickey that spring.

About the time I met Dr. Dickey, I attended a five-day conference that IIN held in Long Beach, California. They'd been publicizing this mega conference from the time I began the program. All the women in my study group from Austin were planning to attend. We would fly together, room together, eat together, and learn together. The months since we'd started the program had flown by so quickly! Before I knew it, it was time to go to the conference. I was so excited! I packed my gear, met my gal pals at the airport, and off we went.

On the first day of the conference, we walked over to the convention center together. Hundreds of people were lining up at the various entrances. We checked in, received our lanyards and nametags, and entered the large stadium-like arena to find our seats. I couldn't believe the number of people there! The convention center was filled with current IIN students and alumni, 4,000 to 5,000 people.

The convention commenced with Joshua Rosenthal, the founder of IIN, addressing the crowd. He had a cheerleader-like presence: positive, full of energy, and enthusiastic. He talked about the future of health coaching, complimenting us for our desire to make this world a better place by following our passion to change the current health care system. "We are the future," he said. "Together, our voices and our knowledge will make an impact. We are a movement and we are creating change together." We gave him a standing ovation.

Joshua spoke several times during the convention. In addition, motivational speakers, successful alumni from IIN, famous authors, personalities, and lecturers from our classes took the stage. Names such as Geneen Roth, Mark Sisson, David Wolfe, and John Robbins addressed the crowd. Several alumni—chefs, product developers, and cookbook authors—spoke about their current projects.

Others had launched their own podcasts and food subscription services—several of which I had recognized or heard of. The list was overwhelming and impressive. At the conclusion of each day's sessions, I felt alive and awake with energy. I thought about all the opportunities to help others heal. I dreamt about maybe one day sharing my story in a convention center filled with thousands of people, becoming a source of inspiration for others as these alumni had been for me.

During the conference, I kept bumping into one particular woman who intrigued me. She was thin, very muscular with a similar build to mine. I thought perhaps she was a runner. She looked like someone who might share common interests—she *was* at the conference after all. I would see her at the conference center, walking the streets of Long Beach on the way home from the conference, and in the elevator at the hotel, which was kind of weird since there were several hotels in the area where attendees were staying. Sometimes she was by herself. Other times she was walking slowly, escorting an older woman to her seat. I finally broke the ice and said something to her when we were both downstairs waiting for the elevator.

"Did you just come back from a run?" I asked.

She smiled. "Yes. It's so beautiful along the coastline. I love the fresh air and the scenery. Did you run out there too?"

"No. My roommate and I took a stroll along the path down to the park. I used to run but don't much anymore." I wanted to tell her why I didn't run, and find out why, for someone who could have been my twin, she was able to keep running. Did she have pain or cramping during her runs? Elimination issues afterwards? She was a health coach, I gathered. Maybe she knew something I didn't, some critical information that would help me heal. I had this strange feeling that she did.

The elevator door opened and she exited. "See you around," she said as the doors shut.

Crap, I said to myself. *Why didn't you ask for her website? Her experience? Augggghhhh!* Frustrated, I walked back to my room to take a shower and get ready for the final day of the conference.

On Monday morning, before we left for the airport, I went down to the hotel gym to ride the bike. When I entered the gym, I looked around, and there she was, running on the treadmill. *Holy shit. This is fo' shizzle the Universe speaking. The conference is over, we've both come to the gym at the same time. We're the only ones here. It's a sign.*

I smiled as I got myself situated on a bike.

After a couple of minutes, she took out her earbuds and motioned my way. "Where are you from?"

For the next twenty minutes, we talked. I shared my story with her and she shared hers with me. She had graduated with the very first IIN class in 1992. Like me, she had digestive issues and used to run marathons and longer distances, but now she only ran a few miles here and there. She described the old days when students used to fly to NY every four to six weeks to study at IIN, before the program became so large that it moved to an online-only learning platform. The older woman she was escorting throughout the conference was Joshua's mother. She had become good friends with Joshua during her time at IIN and helped with some of the office duties when it was just starting out, kind of like his right-hand wo-man. He trusted her and had flown her out to the conference to take care of his mom.

As we talked, she asked me if I was familiar at all with the Landmark Forum. While I'd heard of it, I couldn't remember from whom or in what context. When she began to describe it, I said, "Wait a minute, that's the cult training thing my sister dragged me to several years ago." My sister, acting as my sponsor, had asked me to attend the final day of her workshop and listen to the stories people shared about their experiences. I had no idea what it was, so I went. "It was one of the weirdest things I've ever experienced," I said. "I was so turned off. It felt strange. I didn't connect to it. It felt fake."

She completely understood my strong resistance. "I know exactly how you feel," she said. "It can seem that way from an outsider's perspective, but the actual course is a complete game changer. From what you have told me, I believe you would benefit from attending."

I recalled observing weepy and dramatic performances by recent Landmark graduates, the leader subsequently offering the guests a special promotion to join the next Landmark Forum. Oy! I remember wanting to jail break right then and there, feeling the heebie-jeebies as I glanced across the room at the guests embracing their sponsors, teary-eyed together, signing up to join them in this quest to become renewed, recreated, reinvented. Halla-effing-luyah! It reminded me of the shows I used to watch on Sunday mornings as a kid before the cartoons came on, when the evangelical pastors preached to their congregations. I didn't want to offend Karen, so I told her I had to head out to pick up my kids from school. And that was my one and only experience with Landmark.

But as my doppelgänger described the course after I told her about my experience, it totally and completely felt like something I needed. Especially just after the conference, when I felt a renewed sense of self, very encouraged by what I was learning through IIN. I resonated with so many of the speakers' stories about overcoming difficulties in the face of adversity, and was fascinated as they proceeded to share them with thousands of people. Attending this conference inspired me and motivated me to keep listening and gathering information. The suggestion to attend Landmark was the piece I needed to stay the course and move forward in the right direction.

My new friend described how Landmark was such a game changer for her, even more so than IIN. It transformed her thinking, her way of life, and her professional direction. She'd even gone through additional training to become an advisor to new students. "Please look into this, Ellen," she said. "From what you've told me, I believe this is exactly what you need right now. If there are any questions you have, please feel free to reach out. Find out when there is a forum in your area. They offer them frequently. I suggest that you ride this wave of energy from the conference and sign up as soon as you can." At that point I thanked her profusely, took the contact information she offered, and headed back to my room to shower and set off for the airport.

When I got into the cab, I immediately looked up the Landmark Forum and called to find out the deets. "As a matter of fact," the woman said, "there's a three-day training in Austin beginning this Friday." My heart jumped. This was a sign, *the* sign. I knew I had met that woman for a reason. I knew I needed to do this. I was energized, excited, and terrified. I absolutely, positively *had* to take this course. The one that started just three days after I returned from my five-day IIN getaway. The course, she explained, was three full days. It began at 9 a.m. sharp on Friday (check-in began at 8) and finished up around 10 p.m., but depending on the moderator and the activity, it could last until midnight.

On the plane flying home, and in the cab from the airport, I kept wondering how in the hell I would get Mark to go along with my plan. How would I be able to convince him that this was something I had to do? It was calling to me so powerfully I could feel my insides pulling apart. It would take some planning. First, I needed to play catch up from the days I'd been away. Then, I would have to figure out extra care for the kids. I knew it wasn't an impossible task. Still, I told the woman at Landmark that I would go online and register the minute I got home. And after I talked with Mark, that's what I planned to do.

When I got home, I had a huge knot in my stomach. I felt refreshed and excited to see Mark and the kids. I was also experiencing an inner freak out about asking Mark to fly solo again that weekend. While Mark was curious to hear all about the conference, I could only talk about going through the Landmark Forum. That Friday.

He was exhausted from taking care of the kids and shouldering the extra responsibility while I was away. The last thing he wanted to hear about were my plans for another three-day escape. He wasn't at all pleased *and* actually looked highly annoyed and flabbergasted as I requested another departure from my parental duties. I told him that it was hard for me to explain, that it was something I knew I *had* to do.

Despite Mark's apprehension, I took my laptop and went into the office to sign up. My bullheaded, strong-willed personality was rearing its head again, but this time it wasn't pushing against pain, it was pulling me to act on this hunch, this instinct, this intuition I could sense deep within.

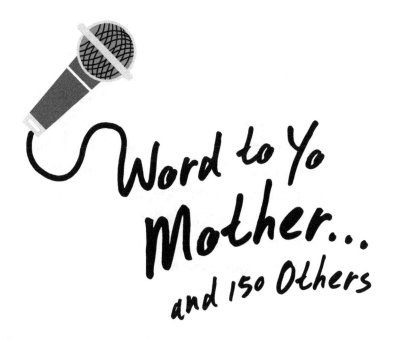

Word to Yo Mother... and 150 Others

THREE DAYS LATER at 9 a.m. sharp, the Landmark Forum orientation began. I approached the auditorium where I would be spending a solid forty-plus hours over the next three days. While waiting my turn in line to register, I couldn't help but people watch, looking over my left shoulder, then my right. Did I recognize anyone? No, thank goodness. I was questioning whether the faces in the crowd looked like "my people." Hmmm, I wasn't quite sure yet.

After receiving my folder and the lanyard with my nametag, I nudged my way through the crowd and chose a seat in one of the middle rows, with a vacant chair on either side. I plastered a smile on my face, turned, and watched as people filtered in. I started to get that uneasy queasy feeling in my stomach that I got when I'd made a rash decision. Did I really want to spend another three full days away from my family? Three days with a bunch of strangers who had only a vague idea of what they were getting themselves into? I sat there, arms crossed, stomach anxious. *Three freakin' days! I should have trusted the instincts I had about this course initially.*

After everyone settled in, our course leader, Sarah, walked up to the podium and introduced herself. Then she turned around and started drawing concentric circles on the whiteboard behind the podium. Pointing to each circle, one by one, she described how we shape our lives and our belief systems. "This circle represents what we were taught to believe," she said. "This circle represents how our experiences in the world have shaped us. This circle represents who we truly are, at our very core without any outside influences, experiences or events in our lives." She gave examples of the types of experiences that could have shaped our realities—being fired from a job, going through divorce, sexual assault, verbal abuse. She was very animated, energetic, and dramatic. So much passion . . . too much passion. *A bit theatrical*, I thought. It kind of weirded me out. I was half paying attention, half checking out the other people in the room.

Some of the attendees had taken the course before, and Sarah asked for a few volunteers to stand up and share their experiences. A man in the back of the room, probably in his late thirties, stood up to share. He began his story and immediately started crying, then full on bawled as he continued, pausing to dry his tears with the wad of Kleenex a volunteer brought to him. He ended with, "This course changed my life. I'm going through the course again to gain more strength and a deeper perspective."

After he sat down, a woman stood up. She started crying before she even began to speak. This course had changed her life too. She shared her transformative tale. One after the other, graduates came forward, grown men and women, totally breaking down, telling horrible, horrible stories about being molested as a child, beaten by their husband, or verbally abused. Each stating, through tears, that this course had changed their lives.

I wondered if these people were hired to "perform" at each of the initial meetings. Maybe they were actresses and actors on the side? The emotional purges were starting to make me feel uncomfortable. Should I pretend to go to the bathroom and quickly bee-line through the nearest exit? If I waited until the break to speak to an admin and tell him or her that I felt uncomfortable and this course wasn't a good fit for me, would I be allowed to leave and get a full refund? A partial refund?

Landmark has been offering the course for more than twenty years. At least 2.4 million people, maybe more, have completed the Forum. Something like 94 percent of graduates polled report that it was a life-changing experience. My sister said it was life-changing. My doppel-ganger from the IIN conference said it was life-changing. The people who'd stood up and shared said it was life-changing. While I probably should have felt compassion, been moved by their cathartic revelations, all I could think was, *What in the hell? Why am I here?* It felt awk-ward to me, and I was afraid I had made the wrong decision to attend.

I looked down at my schedule. It felt incredibly regimented. Each day was broken into five segments. Different subjects for each day, with names like Freedom from Anxiety, How Identities Get Constructed, The Pervasive Influence of the Past. Sarah was explain-ing that the idea of the course is to extract your persona from the stories you've told yourself as a result of the experiences you've had in your life. Maybe you've gone through some terrible trauma and you believe the world isn't safe. Or you lost your father when you were young and believe every man you love will leave you. Or a parent or coach always said, "You can do better than that," so you never think you're good enough.

After orientation, we started our first segment. I decided to stick with it because some of what Sarah was saying started to make sense. The less drama, the more I tuned in. I began to appreciate her energy and the knowledge she shared. More people came forward to speak about those life experiences that had created their story. Day turned into night as we continued to discuss topics that create the feelings, emotions, and beliefs that cause us strife, anxiety, conflict, and concern in our lives. We learned that we linger in that space of conflicted and painful emotions and create stories about ourselves that we believe are true. These stories are based on those traumatic circumstances, and spark the internal dialogue that affects how we move through life.

As I listened to people's stories, something clicked. It ceased to matter what their story was. It became my story too. One and the same. It was true for all of us. Each person in that room felt those emotions and related to the stories being shared. These experiences and personal narratives all had common threads. We began to see that most of what we believe about ourselves is made up—fiction—with common elements we all share that affect how we move through life.

During each segment, we were assigned a task that aligned with the theme or topic we were working on. Once, we had to go up to someone else in the group and tell them a story. When we discussed our parents and the environment in which we were raised, there was a long discussion about our mothers and how their influence has such a profound influence on our personas. Several people had to clear energy or communication issues with mothers before they could move forward, so after lunch on the second day, our assignment was to make a phone call to our mothers.

I went out to the parking lot, got into my car, closed the door, cracked the window, and clutching a paper on which I'd scribbled some notes about what I was going to say, I called my mom. She answered the phone, and, voice shaking, I said, "Hi, Mom. I'm in the middle of a class and I'm calling you to discuss our relationship. I want to move forward so we don't have any more hurt feelings, any more strife." I took a deep breath. "Please, I want you to hear me out."

"Okay, sure, Ellen," she said. "You know I love you."

"I know that my actions don't always or may not frequently align with yours."

She said nothing, just let me talk.

I started crying, and I don't cry or show emotion very often. "Please respect that I'm an individual. I'm an adult. I love you very much, too, and cannot thank you and Dad enough for raising me and putting up with so much of my ornery bullshit growing up. I know I wasn't an easy one to raise. The life path I follow and the choices I make may not always follow the same trajectory as yours. But that doesn't matter. They intersect at several points along the way. I just need you to acknowledge that and not judge me. I want you to know that I have so much respect for you and Dad and that I love you both dearly. I feel so fortunate that we're in Austin together and that however I choose to raise, feed, or educate my children, you're here sharing those experiences with us. It means so much to me."

The conversation lasted almost forty minutes. She said she had enjoyed speaking to me and was thankful for my call. I thought she'd heard what I had to say and appreciated my honesty and sincere desire to reach out and clear whatever cloudy air had been floating between us. After I hung up, I definitely felt better.

On the last morning of class, before I left the house, Mark and I went out for an early morning walk. I told him I knew I could be a better partner, a better mother, a better friend. "There are a lot of things I do that upset you. I don't always give you my 100 percent attention, I'm never on time. I don't always eat with the family. I want to change all that."

I poured out my heart, telling him how things were going to change. "This class has really proved to me that my actions can have a tremendous impact on the people I love the most. I haven't been paying attention to my actions, not recognizing the impact of my behaviors. I want to show you and the kids more respect. I want to be on time. I will work hard to make that happen and to eat with you all as a family." As I spoke these words to Mark, a subtle shift occurred. I was discovering that when I'm brave enough to speak my voice and share my true emotions, I feel much stronger. This was such a change from constantly feeling afraid and worried about what others might be thinking. I also felt that after I communicated with both Mark and my mother, they too felt more open, accepting, and willing to share with me.

On the final day of the Forum, we spent the entire time discussing how everything, all our beliefs, stem from fear, whether it's fear of speaking out, fear of relationships, fear of commitment—fear triggers all negative emotional response and is therefore attached to *all* the limiting or negative stories we create. I started reflecting on the fear of sharing my feelings with my mother and Mark. *Why am I so afraid to voice my emotions to those I love the most? Why is it so hard to express my weaknesses, insecurities, and desire for a deeper connection?* And my lifelong fear of never being able to achieve the high expectations I set for myself. *Why can't I just go out and have fun and not be all caught up in my head?* I wondered. *Why am I so fearful of not measuring up? Of not being good enough?* I thought about all my races, triathlons, marathons. Was Nike barking up my tree to become my sponsor? To offer me their gear and outfit me for all my races? Um, not exactly. Then why in the heck was I insisting that I achieve, attain, and improve my goals, time and time and time again? I realized I had nothing to prove to anyone—including myself.

Sarah explained in numerous ways that we're all trying to separate from the fear associated with our past experiences so we can create new possibilities for ourselves. I wanted to stand up and share, but I couldn't quite make myself. As I continued to hear new stories, see new faces emerge, and relate my personal struggles with theirs, the urge to share my story intensified. Before I knew it and could stop myself, I stood up, walked over to the closest mic, and, heart pounding, voice shaking, I shared. I started out slowly, talking about my exercise addiction, my food issues that began way back in high school. As I spoke, the words started to roll off my tongue. I talked about how I always pushed myself to perform, excel, and be the best, and how much internal pressure and stress that created. I shared how I was constantly competing with myself and if I didn't consistently improve, I regarded my performance as a failure. I wasn't good enough. On the outside, I was perceived as a great athlete—fit, healthy, and strong—but my stoic facade masked the weakness and fear inside.

It was the first time I said out loud, in public, that I had any issues with exercise or food. And it was in front of 150 people to boot! I kept my shit together at first, though as I listened to my own voice describe how hard I had been on myself my entire life, as the words resonated, I started to feel that sensation of my throat closing, my heart beating out of my chest, and my eyes welled with tears. Then, I officially lost it. I can't even remember what I said. I was in another zone, scared shitless, shaking inside but somehow also serene.

When I finished speaking, I still felt scared, vulnerable, and humiliated that I had been dealing with these issues. I couldn't believe that I had just made them public to an auditorium filled with 150 fellow forum freaks. I was overcome with a sense of shame and embarrassment. *Why had I shared all that? What had possessed me to tell a room full of complete strangers what I hadn't even completely admitted to myself? Augggghhhh!* I'd fallen prey to Landmark's scheme. I'd caved. I, too, had joined the cult, drunk the Kool-Aid. *What a fool you are!* I said to myself. It was the lack of sleep and emotional drainage talking, I decided. I'd been *brainwashed*!!! I kept my eyes on the carpet in front of me as I sniffed and sulked back to my chair. I was sure people were thinking that I was fucked up in the head, that I had all these issues—how obvious it was by the looks of me. I probably hadn't told them anything they couldn't see for themselves.

We had a break shortly after my "performance." I got up to stretch my legs and go outside for a breath of fresh air. I took my phone so I could isolate myself and look down at the screen instead of having to make eye contact with anyone. But on my way out the door, all these people, mainly women, came up to me, saying, "That was amazing." "What you just shared was awesome." "I've been through that, too." And, "You've gained the strength to talk about this." Women told me that they'd struggled or were struggling with similar fears and frustrations about coming up short of their own expectations, setting extremely high bars for how they needed to look, act, or perform.

Many admitted to food aversions and addictions to exercise. Others acknowledged that they, too, were struggling with a pressure to succeed that had built up inside them like a balloon about to burst. When I heard what they had to say, every last drop of fear melted away.

Why was I so afraid to share this? I wondered. This was a game changer. Telling my story shifted my emotions. Changed my life. I finally recognized I wasn't the only one wrestling. I wasn't horribly different. I was not alone. There was a community acknowledging my struggle, supporting it, and praising someone like me, someone no one would suspect—the coach, the exercise instructor, the personal trainer, the athlete, the uber volunteer, the ultra-organized mom—was battling these demons every day.

It was a huge relief to speak my truth and feel that my words had created a safe place, an open forum, familiar territory where others could share. Instead of feeling isolated, like a failure or a loser for speaking out, I felt accepted, validated, and recognized as part of a community. One where people were commending me for

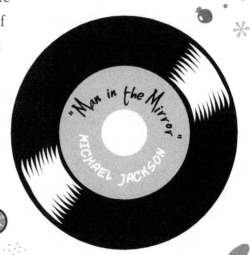

my honesty and bravery. I was not alone. That was exactly when I realized that sharing my experiences, my trials and tribulations, and being frank and truthful about my journey could potentially help other people.

A few months after finishing the Landmark Forum, I took one of their follow-up, advanced courses. The group met every Thursday evening for six weeks. Each week, we were given small in-class and at-home assignments that we did on our own or with the small group we'd been assigned to. One week, the leader, Carl, wearing his mic, stood in front of the whiteboard, outlining that evening's topic—accomplishing what we set out to do, overcoming obstacles, and how to get out of our own way. We discussed how to accomplish something you want to do when you continuously tell yourself you can't.

Our in-class assignment was to write about an event or experience that shaped our lives for the better, changed the mission of our life's work. While sharing my story during the three-day forum had hugely changed the trajectory of my life, I chose to write about my Universal Intervention, my surgery in March of 2010. After we finished our in-class assignment, we reconvened as a group and used the remainder of the class time to share our work with each other. Carl called on me to read an excerpt from my assignment. Hesitantly, I agreed. I opted to stay in my chair as I read rather than go up on the podium. He was okay with that, although he motioned for me to stand up.

I agreed, stood up, and began reading about my surgery, how much I had learned since then and how I wanted to use this knowledge to help others heal. Carl started dissecting my words, asking specifically how I thought I might be of service to others, how I might be able to apply my knowledge and experience. I looked at him and responded, without thinking. I made a flip comment: "I should write a book."

"Why do you want to write a book?" Carl asked.

"I dunno. I'm just saying that I've gathered so much information throughout my healing process. I have a story to tell. Don't take everything so literally."

Ignoring my comment about being too literal, he said, "Okay. What's your story?" With Landmark, it's always a deep, deep probe. They hook you and then they keep going deeper, deeper, deeper. So he wasn't letting up. He motioned for me to come forward, to join him up on the podium in front of the infamous white board, and converse in depth about the idea of writing a book.

"I've dealt with food issues and exercise addiction," I said. "Then I realized there are lots of people who share those struggles. I've had several gut issues and a major surgery. I've learned a lot, experientially, as I've attempted to heal my gut. I now recognize the relationship between my gut and my brain. As I've recovered my health and my gut issues have begun to improve, I've gained clarity surrounding thoughts about my exercise habits and the types of food I was feeding my body. I'm much more adept at listening to my body's signals with self-compassion. I've become less regimented in my behaviors, and have begun to tap into my intuition, allowing my heart to lead instead of my head. I feel I could write a book about all I've been through. I sense there are a lot of people who can relate to and might benefit from my story, whether it's in their head, their gut, or both."

He didn't miss a beat. "So why don't you?"

"Why don't I what?"

"Write a book."

"I can't write a book. I don't write."

He just looked at me. He wasn't going to let me off that easily. "Okay. I can't *sit down* to write. You've heard me talk during this course. I'm in constant motion. Always. Writing a book is a huge commitment. I wouldn't even know where to begin!"

"Good," he said. "This is good stuff. If you want to write a book, how would you go about achieving that goal?"

"I don't know. I honestly have no idea what's involved. It sounds like a much bigger project or goal than I could ever pull off."

"It's simple, really. Anyone can write a book. You just break it down. You just set yourself up with a series of achievable goals and then determine the ways that you can accomplish those goals, enlisting help and support wherever and whenever you need it. You have a story to tell. Your desire is to help others heal by sharing your experience. This sets you up perfectly with the end goal. There are plenty of people out there who have written books or helped others write books before. Enlist them to help you."

A guy in the back corner of the room raised his hand. "I'm an editor," he said, "and I can help you find somebody to work with to meet that goal."

Then somebody else chimed in. "I can help you find someone too."

People started passing business cards to me. I stood there, dumbfounded at what had just gone down. The charge of excitement about the ownership of writing a book hit me like a shockwave.

I felt that same ownership I'd felt *so many times* after registering for a race, volunteering to chair an event, or sending out an invitation to a party. Once I commit, I do not go back on my word! I own it right then and there and will work tirelessly to accomplish the end goal with whatever resources I can find to support me through the process. I stick to my word and my word sticks to me. Why would writing a book be any different? It was a very familiar process.

That's how it works in the Landmark courses too. You're surrounded by people who support you in achieving your goal, who work from a place of "You can do it!" and teach you to believe in yourself, move forward with your dreams, and not let any of the stories you've carried with you from the past block your path in the future. So, that night, I got into the headspace of "Let's do this. I can do this." The more I thought about it, the more I realized I had to write the book. It all made sense! Suddenly I felt that this was my purpose in life, why I'd come through the surgery and endured everything else on my healing path. I had always been an educator. I educated people about fitness and food. Writing the book was a natural next step.

I will always be grateful to Landmark. Sharing my story in front of 150 people was scary. I proved that when I'm brave enough to expose my flaws, my weaknesses, and my fears, when I am truthful and authentic about who I am and what I stand for, when I lower my own expectations and don't always strive for perfection, I become stronger, more resilient. I build community. I learned that across the board, when we face our own fears, we step into our power, which is greater than any other driving emotion.

The day I shared my story in front of 150 people, I was blown away by how many identified with what I'd said. They were touched and inspired by my strength to come forward. I was amazed that so many faced the same angst, were grappling with their feelings and resisting their fears. I began to wonder how many of us suffer in silence when we could empower and inspire each other to speak our truths, to share our struggles and support one other in the process. I wanted to help. Right then and there, my internal compass registered true north. I wasn't going to hide from myself or anyone else any longer.

Locavore Kicks In

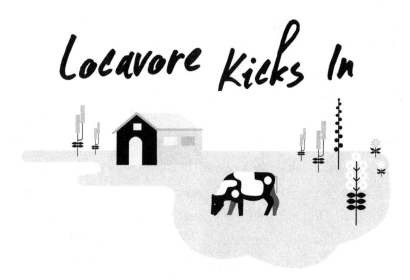

AS I HEALED, I continued to develop a much healthier relationship with food. I also began to enjoy cooking, which I had never made time for up to that point. I collected kitchen gadgets that accelerated and slowed down the cooking process (Vitamix, Crock-Pot, pressure cooker), which I loved to use to create and enhance new flavors and textures in dishes. I became a sponge when it came to learning more about foods that heal and those that steal from your health. It seemed that the roots of the IIN health coach certification were now sprouting. I had always been passionate about clean, organic food, and suddenly, after Landmark, and the investigation into my own healing, I had an overwhelming desire to start spreading the gospel about buying from local farmers. My focus shifted from my personal health to helping others eat locally, seasonally, and sustainably. I especially loved connecting with those who grew the food I ate. I had so much appreciation for their hard work and commitment. Food is fuel, but it's also connection. Food connects us to the earth, to those who grow our food, and to each other.

So I started my business—The Locavore Next Door—offering individual health and wellness coaching, corporate wellness talks, community lectures, school presentations, grocery store tours, farmers market tours, farm field trips, and pantry clean-out. I sort of fell into my business. While I was healing my gut and experimenting with adding animal protein back into my diet, I became hyperaware of where these proteins came from, what the animals ate, and how they were treated and slaughtered. I was on a quest to find out more about how animals were raised for consumption, what they were fed, if they were allowed to roam free in the pasture and bask in the sun. I could only wrap my head around introducing meat back into my diet if I knew that the animals were pure, clean, and humanely treated.

I began traveling to the farmers markets in Austin, interviewing the ranchers who were selling there: "Have you raised these animals yourself? Where is your ranch? Do the animals roam freely on pasture? Do they just eat grass and insects? Do you supplement them with feed? If so, is it GMO feed? Do you spray your land with pesticides? Are the chickens in coops that you move to different parts of the property or are they always eating, pooping, and laying in the same location?"

It was truly an inquisition. But instead of the ranchers being annoyed with my questions, they absolutely loved the chance to talk about their work. They had a tremendous amount of passion and took pride in their profession. They appreciated my curiosity. I learned so much from them while sharing my struggles to improve my health, wanting to accomplish that primarily through the foods I ate. The inquisitions morphed into conversations, which developed into friendships.

For years, twice a week—Wednesday afternoons and Saturday mornings—I hit the local farmers markets to buy produce, eggs, meat, cheeses, canned pickles, and jam from local farmers and artisans. I found an amazing assortment—grown, prepared, and sold by people who clearly loved what they were doing, who had a deep connection with and respect for food and the earth. They were thrilled to talk about varietals, growing conditions, cooking methods, and offer samples—the whole food experience. This food, grown and prepared with love and respect, is what helped me heal and what I wanted people to learn more about and consume more often.

I wanted to help others become aware of how fruits and vegetables are grown, shipped, and stored before reaching their plates. I wanted them to experience the difference in the taste of a fruit or vegetable grown locally and in season versus one that had been harvested before it was ripe then shipped hundreds or thousands of miles to sit in a refrigerated warehouse before being placed on display in the produce aisle. My desire was to teach people the impact their buying decisions had on our environment and explain to them that foods that have just been harvested contain so many more nutrients. Cooking local and seasonal food is simple and straightforward because flavor is the main ingredient, and when purchasing, preparing, and consuming food with these principles in mind, they will experience an improvement in their health.

These farmers and ranchers became more than teachers and acquaintances. They became friends. I was concerned about their land when we had a torrential rain or a hard freeze, and about their bottom line when an infestation of bugs wiped out a crop. This was their life-blood, and nothing, not even Mother Nature, could get in the way of their passion to grow and share the literal fruits of their labor with others. On freezing cold Saturday mornings in the winter, I would purchase bags of hand and feet warmers and distribute them to the vendors who stood outside shivering for hours awaiting the few customers brave enough to face the elements. The shoppers who attended quickly made their rounds and hurried back to their heated cars. The market became my church, a gathering of like-minded people I appreciated, respected, and connected with more than I could have ever imagined.

Nathan Heath was one of the farmers I visited with and bought from each week. He was incredibly passionate about his soil, his farming methods. I went out with my family to visit his farm and helped him clear land for planting. He and his mom took us on a tour. They were clearly proud of their farmland. They raised earthworms, millions of them, which increase the amount of air and water in the soil. Their castings serve as a type of fertilizer. I saw the amazing compost pile they maintained, which added valuable nutrients back into their soil.

I learned so much in our weekly conversations. Nathan was well read and introduced me to the writings of Wendell Berry, a novelist and farmer in Kentucky, and Will Allen, a retired professional basketball player turned farmer and founder of Growing Power, an urban farm in Milwaukee. One day at the market, Nathan talked to me about his life goals. "I don't only want to farm as a business, I want to create future farmers, good farmers, farmers who understand how to farm."

I was so excited by what he was saying. I wanted to help!

"I want to build a space on my farm that can house interns," he said, "an educational community room, and a commercial kitchen, so we can teach our farmers how to cook the produce they're planting and harvesting, and how to prepare these foods to bring out their optimal flavor. I want to bring chefs and store managers to tour the farm so that farmers can embrace all aspects of farm to table and gain a better understanding of how the chefs are using our produce in their dishes. Farmers and chefs can collaborate on the best items to grow, which varietals of an onion or a tomato or a green would be most desirable. I also want to start hosting dinners out on my farm with local chefs, educating the end consumer about what we grow and how we operate."

I could see the fire in his eyes, and I caught his enthusiasm. "I'm going to help you do that."

"What?" He looked puzzled by my announcement.

"I'll help you raise the money," I said. "We'll do a Kickstarter, an online crowdfunding campaign. We'll get the media involved. We'll have a kick-off event where we'll introduce the campaign. People will donate what they can—$5, $50, $500. We'll invite everyone we know who might be interested." My mind raced, firing ideas a mile a minute. I felt such a strong desire to help him fulfil his dream. I knew I could make this happen. After all the events I had organized?

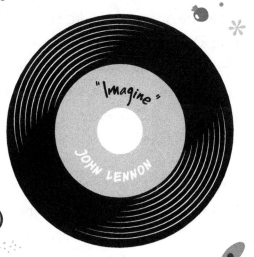

One of the things I loved to do and did very well was to connect people.

I've always had a knack for bringing people together. I'm a good listener and can hear what people need—when they feel stuck, have a position to fill, or need assistance in an area and don't know where to turn. I have a keen sense of filling that void. Since starting my business, I've connected chefs with farmers and ranchers, bakers with restaurants, fitness junkies with functional medicine doctors, and small business owners with CEOs. I feel that in addition to teaching people how to move their bodies to improve their health, my place in this world is to introduce people to local food, local farms, and local businesses. All I had to do was convince Nathan to dig it—my idea, not his soil.

I knew we could raise the money. I started thinking out loud about whom we could approach. Between the chefs at some of the restaurants Nathan sold to and some of the people I knew from the markets, local food organizations, and nonprofits, we had the potential to make the event a huge success and to get Nathan's funding. He held up his hand to stop me. He didn't want me to do it. "It's a lot of work. It will be a lot of trouble and will take a long time."

I heard the hesitancy in his voice, but I kept at it. "No, no, we can really do this. We can make it happen." My enthusiasm and unwillingness to back down finally wore Nathan out. I have a knack for that too, as I have had a lot of practice with Mark. Finally, he agreed and we got to work.

One of the restaurants I had in mind to host the event had a beautiful open space and back patio. The owner, Shawn Cirkiel, an exceptionally generous, super nice guy and huge supporter of local farms, had several restaurants in town and purchased regularly from Nathan. I approached him and said, "Hey, I'm thinking about doing a Kickstarter campaign for Nathan, and I want to host a kickoff event with a panel discussion about the future of farming. I want to invite chefs, foragers, and farmers to participate." I told him we'd invite people to purchase tickets, listen to the panel, and donate to the Kickstarter campaign. We'd serve food and drink, using produce from Nathan's farm. "Would you consider doing that?" Without blinking an eye, Shawn agreed, and we started planning.

At that point, I had a chef, a farmer, and a venue. Nathan put me in touch with a forager, Valerie, who worked at a local hotel. She was extremely well-connected to the local farmers and ranchers and sourced local produce and proteins for the hotel's restaurant. She would learn the availability of items from local farms and supply that information to the hotel chefs so they could plan their menus accordingly. She agreed to participate in the event and the panel, and was instrumental in helping to bring on other chefs and restauranteurs to join her.

I also reached out to the original Austin locavore, Jesse Griffiths. He owned a food truck, Dai Due, which served breakfast at the farmers market every Saturday morning. Everything he offered was made from only locally sourced ingredients. He hunted with local ranchers, fished with the local fishermen. He was purchasing from Austin's local farms more than a decade prior to the farm-to-table movement coming into vogue. He would talk to the farmers about what they were planting and when it would be harvested and go to the farms to pick and buy produce. His dishes were amazing and people would line up early to order his daily offerings before they sold out, which they always did.

To preserve the local bounty, he started canning, selling pickles and mustards, fermenting cabbage to make sauerkraut and peppers to make his own hot sauces. He made amazing charcuterie—sausage, pâtés, and the *best* chicken liver mousse. The first time I decided to branch out and indulge in eating organ meat (I had been reading about how beneficial it was to my health), I almost freaked out. Not only was it delicious, but I could actually feel my body absorb it. It felt like my system was thanking me for filling a void that had been empty for so long. I began to crave it. It was as if the wholesome, pure ingredients had medicinal qualities. People lined up to buy these items too. Jesse created and spearheaded the locavore movement in Austin. He lived it, ate it, breathed it.

Nathan is a very well-respected farmer and sells to many of the best restaurants in Austin. The chefs know of the superb quality and care he takes with his farm. One chef, Bryce Gilmore, whose dad has been in the business for a long time and has always been a friend and big supporter of all the local farms, agreed to participate. He started a wildly successful food truck, Odd Duck Farm to Trailer, which he had eventually closed to open a small brick and mortar farm-to-table restaurant, Barley Swine. He was getting a huge amount of recognition, including being nominated (the first in a string of consecutive nominations) for the James Beard award, Best Chef in the Southwest Region. His menu changes daily, depending on what's available locally. There is always an extremely creative blend of flavors, tastes, and textures in each dish. Another chef in Bryce's restaurant, Sam Hellman-Mass, joined the panel as well.

The final piece was to find someone to moderate the panel discussion. The editor-publisher of *Edible Austin* magazine, Marla Camp, was my first choice. We met for lunch to discuss the event. I explained what we were trying to accomplish—not only raising money for Nathan to add an educational component to his farm but to inform the community about the necessity of supporting the future generation of farmers. She had moderated panels for several different events in town and conducted several interviews with famous chefs and cookbook authors. She was the perfect fit. She didn't hesitate one bit. "Sure, I'd love to," she said, as she took another sip of her tea.

The event turned out to be a huge success. We announced the Kickstarter, gave everyone the link to donate to the campaign, and after the event, the word spread. Within a few weeks, the campaign was fully funded. Nathan got his money and was able to construct the first phase of his project—a building that would provide housing to a farm intern and a classroom where educational discussions about farming would be held. I felt so positive about supporting somebody I really, truly believed was doing the right thing.

After that event, I continued to immerse myself in the local food scene, supporting farmers, ranchers, and locally sourcing chefs. I became involved in the Slow Food movement, eventually joining the board of the Austin chapter. I helped to lobby for the sale of raw milk (which has yet to pass in Texas) and the future of Urban Farms in Austin. I facilitated fundraising events, taught classes, coached private clients, and continued to connect people. It provided nourishment on all levels—body, mind, heart, and soul.

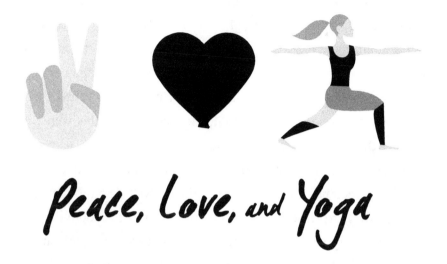

Peace, Love, and Yoga

MY APPROACH TO EXERCISE had also transformed. The concept of fueling my body on a more metaphorical level—with passion versus results-driven anxiety and stress—was now manifesting. Yoga became my lifesaver. I swapped the love of adrenaline for a deeper intensity, a sense of connection, groundedness, and the spirituality I craved. Yoga allowed me to move and breathe simultaneously, to send breath to every cell, to feel an association between my mind and my body. It created an awareness that I otherwise might not have been able to tap into.

I'd been doing yoga for years, but never with the awareness and devotion I had after Landmark. What drew me to my mat in the first place, although I hadn't realized it before, was the message, the intention, and the transparency of the instructors. I connected with them, but on a very different level from those trainers and instructors I worked with at the gym.

These yoga instructors were raw and real; the intention they set for each class reflected the personal struggles and triumphs they were experiencing. Before class started, they would sit down on their mats in the front of the room and share what was going on in their lives—divorce, financial strain, love, or loss. The stories they told were personal, with a universal point, addressing what the struggle was about, why they might be going through it, and the emotions that were presenting themselves at that moment. They would admit if they were holding on to fear, resisting change, or overcoming conflict as they sought to become more accepting of themselves. The thoughts and feelings they expressed touched every person in the room, stirring emotions every student could relate to. The experience was similar to Landmark. The stories were all different but the emotional battles were the same. I embraced the whole experience. The practice was an expression of peace, unity, and strength from the inside out—all elements I needed to reintegrate as I became my whole self again.

Unlike the bootcamps, spin classes, and cardio-crushing workouts I was used to taking and teaching, there were no disguises, no fronts, no "Are you ready to get your ass kicked and handed to you on a silver platter" persona. The game-day face I sported along with the "woot-woots" I yelled and screamed over the mic at the top of my lungs were uncharacteristic and unfamiliar in yoga. When I taught a class, that's who I had to show up as, it's what I was known for, and those expectations incited my performance. Even if I felt small some days, or sad or weak or tired, it didn't matter. As the stereo went on and the playlist queued up, the real me faded away and almost immediately morphed into my fitness façade. This is how I approached *every single class.*

I gravitated toward more challenging yoga classes, but I also sought out instructors whose stories I could relate to. I got stronger—physically, mentally, spiritually. Yoga fed my soul, fed that desire to connect with myself on a deeper level, to take in this community of instructors and students who were sharing their authentic selves with me. I attribute a lot of my healing to yoga. My yoga practice is a huge, huge part of who I am and what I love. It's community. It's my foundation. It's balance. It's breath. It's awareness. I wouldn't be whole without it.

After Landmark, it took me a while to find a practice I aligned with. I was a yoga whore, hopping in and out of studios all over Austin. All different styles—Bikram, Vinyasa flow, Hatha, Iyengar—I tried many different teachers at several different studios. I followed some teachers around, became part of their tribe. I talked to friends and other fitness buffs about where they practiced and which classes they enjoyed the most. Upon numerous recommendations, I bought an introductory special at a studio I had never been to before. As I was checking out the studio's website, I saw they offered a Mysore-style Ashtanga class. I had never tried Ashtanga, let alone Mysore style. The two-hour time frame worked perfectly with my schedule, so I called them before class one day, asking what Mysore was all about.

"It's a self-practice," said the woman who answered the phone. "You're taught a series of postures, or asanas, in a very specific sequence, with a very specific alignment to each posture—all movements tied to your breath count."

It sounded intriguing, new, and exciting! I raced over to give it a try. I walked into the studio and introduced myself to the teacher. She told me to just observe, and after she led the class in the chant and checked in with the other students, she'd give me a set of postures to work on. I followed her into a small room where six others were practicing independently, all different levels. Some postures looked familiar. Others I didn't recognize; they looked quite challenging. When the students saw the instructor—they stopped what they were doing and came to stand at the top of their mats as she called out, Samasthiti.

She began chanting loudly in Sanskrit and every few words she would pause and repeat the phrase and the others in the room would chant along with her: "vande gurūṇāṃ caraṇāravinde sandarśita svātma sukhāvabodhe niḥśreyase jāṅgalikāyamāne saṃsāra hālāhala mohaśāntyai ābāhu puruṣākāraṃ śaṅkhacakrāsi dhāriṇam sahasra śirasam śvetaṃ praṇamāmi patañjalim. Om." Everyone Om'd together, then returned to practicing the postures they'd been so focused on.

I watched in amazement as one woman wound a leg behind her head and pressed her palms together at her heart in prayer position. Another guy folded himself in half, head pushed between his legs, ears clamped between his knees, arms wound around his body and clasped behind his back. He started walking—five steps forward and then five steps back. Another—body facing one direction, head and neck another—was twisted and bound so tight that I couldn't even figure out which arm or leg was connected to which shoulder or hip. All the students seemed so internally motivated; I noted their extreme focus, the concentration in their eyes. I listened to the steadiness of their breath while they moved from one posture to the next. Holy crap! They're so strong! How are they doing these postures? I felt that familiar rush of a challenge. This is awesome.

The instructor came over to help me get started. "Do five sun salutations A. Use your Ujjayi breath, inhale through the nose and exhale audibly through the nose. I want to hear your breath." Then she went to check on other students.

A few minutes later, I finished, and stood waiting. *That was easy enough.* The instructor saw that I had completed the sun salutations, and called out, "Now five sun salutations B." I started in. When I went into Warrior I, she came over and grabbed my hip. "Pull your hip back. Place your foot there. Square off your shoulders. There's a very specific alignment for each Ashtanga posture. You need to master that." She kept watching me as I went through my sun Bs, adjusting my form every so often. Everyone else was moving though postures that seemed unfamiliar and looked rather difficult. They were sweating profusely, breathing heavily. It was hard to keep my eyes off them and focus on what I was doing.

After thirty-five minutes of sun salutations, the instructor said, "Okay, that's great. Take shavasana."

What?! It was a two-hour class. I'd barely started. *Did I flunk the audition?*

"Come back tomorrow," she said. "Repeat what you did today. If you get it right—the right *drishti* (fixed gaze), the right breath—then we'll move on, add more."

I lay on my mat, eyes closed, pretending to focus on my breath, disappointed. My time in the class had been short and not very challenging. I contemplated going to another yoga class later that afternoon so I could get in a decent workout.

On the way home, I gave myself a pep talk: *Yoga is all about the journey. Be patient. Just stick with it, and you'll get there. Everything takes practice. Don't rush the process.*

I went back the next day. The instructor gave me a few more

postures. I moved further into the series. I began to fall in love with the practice. I felt so excited. During the workouts with my trainer Mark, I told him about my Ashtanga practice, and demonstrated some of the new postures I was learning. I explained how the series moved from standing to seated, and all the way through to the finishing sequence. "We'll have to keep working on my core. It's *all* in the core." I was so excited to tell him when I advanced in the series. "I got a new posture!" I'd say as soon as I walked through the door. It was a big deal, an accomplishment. I was moving forward at a good pace. The sequence was challenging, and I loved it.

One morning during our session, Mark told me that Dr. Dickey, who I was still seeing, had just brought on a functional medicine doc from Dallas to work with him. "Here's the really interesting part," Mark said. "His wife, Priya, is an Ashtanga yoga teacher."

That got my attention. "What? You're kidding." I was so intrigued. There are so few teachers, so few studios that offer Ashtanga because such a small number of people practice it compared to the other styles of yoga. When I got home, I googled Priya's website and watched her videos. She was incredibly strong. She had trained in Mysore, India, with guru Shri R. Sharath Jois, the son of K. Pattabhi Jois, the Indian yoga teacher who developed Ashtanga yoga.

I contacted her immediately and told her I wanted to take private lessons when she was settled in Austin. She arrived a couple of weeks later and I began working with her in an upstairs room of the house where Dr. Dickey's Holistic Family Medicine practice and Mark's studio were located. I was her first student. She impressed me from the get-go—a phenomenal teacher, incredibly passionate and patient. She was intelligent, perceptive, respectful of my character, determination, and energy. We had very similar personalities. She could relate to me. And I could relate to her. She consulted with Dr. Dickey (with my permission), who told her everything there was to know about me: "She's very driven. You better watch her. She's going to want to excel very quickly. She's very strong, but she's also very strong-willed. And she'll push herself beyond her limits if needed . . ."

Priya took into account Dr. Dickey's description of me and progressed me in a challenging yet mindful manner. I wasn't pushing myself too hard but was very focused and involved in my practice, which accelerated quickly since we were working together one-on-one, usually four to five days a week. When we weren't together, I practiced on my own. I completely stopped going to the studio where I had learned a large part of the primary series. In Ashtanga, you're only supposed to work with one teacher. They are *your teacher*. You are *their student*. I was committed to Priya and she to me. It was a perfect pairing. She had been trained by the guru in Mysore, and I wanted to learn everything the proper way.

Ashtanga provided me with the physical challenge I craved. It forced me to focus on my breath in each pose, caused me to stay uberfocused on the sequence, my *drishti*, and attentive to balancing out my body by working through both standing and seated postures, twists, forward folds, and backbends. But I didn't want to let go of my other exercise modalities. I continued my sessions with Mark because I loved lifting weights and the sessions made me look and feel healthier and stronger. I had also started going to Lagree Fitness classes, a forty-five minute workout on a machine called a Megaformer. It's a total body workout, a ton of core—more effective and efficient than anything I'd experienced in my twenty-plus years in the fitness industry.

"I love Lagree," I told Priya. "It's making me stronger in my yoga practice." So between my weights, Lagree, and Ashtanga I had plenty of variety, lots of intensity, and felt as though they complimented each other beautifully. This was the first time I recognized that I didn't miss the running, the pounding, the impact. I felt stronger from my center, both mentally and physically. I could see changes in my body, my strength, and I felt more clarity and mindfulness around exercise.

When I first began Ashtanga, the teacher told me it could take up to five years to get through the full primary series, maybe even longer. When I heard that I thought, *Five years? You've got to be kidding! I'll get it all within a year.* And that's exactly what happened. After starting Mysore at the studio and practicing for six months with Priya, she started me on the second, or intermediate, series of postures. I was excited, feeding off each progression. Being given another pose was like a gift; I felt such a sense of worth, accreditation, accomplishment. It changed the outlook of my entire day.

I worked hard, for both of us. It was really challenging and I loved that. Once I completed a posture fully, really mastered it, she would add another, then another. Sometimes Priya held me in a posture for weeks at a time, if not months, before she allowed me to move on. When I stayed in one place for a long time, it seemed like an eternity. In the traditional Ashtanga practice, you're only allowed to advance to the next posture when you're told by your teacher that you're ready. It can bring up feelings of frustration, anger, and impatience. The teacher takes many factors into account before he or she grants the student another posture. If the instructor sees that the student is too anxious or agitated about not progressing, the teacher may use this as an opportunity to utilize the yoga sutras, or principles, to help silence the fluctuations of the mind. Or they may see that the student's ego is wrapped up in the pose and choose to hold them there until that sense of selfishness fades away. They might also feel that the student is pushing too hard to get to the next posture. This, too, can be a teaching tool for the student to soften his or her practice, breathe more fully, and embrace patience and gratitude before moving along.

At some point, as the student masters more postures, the teacher will drop postures from the previous sequence, but I hadn't quite reached that point. Every day, I'd complete the entire primary sequence and then begin the second series before embarking on the finishing, or closing, sequence (which usually lasted about twenty minutes). My practice was running one and a half to two hours long. Every minute was intense. I challenged myself to perform to the level I'd achieved the previous day. If I could complete a pose fully one day, I expected to do it again the next time I came to my mat. And so I went on down that rabbit hole . . . once again. Even when my body was telling me, *I can't hold the posture*, and Priya,

seeing my exhaustion, told me I could move more quickly through the posture, that I didn't have to hold it for five breaths, I'd push through anyway. Five breaths was the ideal. Five breaths was standard, traditional. Five breaths would make it perfect. *I don't want to cheat myself or my teacher*, I thought.

When I made it to my final posture in the series, the one we had been working to improve, to progress, I was exhausted, but I'd keep at it. Typically, you're supposed to attempt a posture two to three times, and then let it go, not dwell on it, but I ignored that rule. "Let's move on," Priya would say after my third try, and I'd say, "No, no, no. I'm soooo close. Just one more time. I think I can get it." My adrenaline would overtake my exhaustion, I'd be hell bent on getting it. She'd usually succumb to my pleas and flash me a crooked smile because we were truly two peas in a pod. I was like a kid wanting one more story. I'd say, "Just one more time. One more." Completely ignoring the voice inside saying, *I'm tired. I'm drained. I don't want to do this. I can't do this. I don't like this pose.* But I kept at it—two hours a day, four days a week.

Priya and I had worked together for close to a year when she was preparing to leave for India to study with her guru for three months. I felt exhausted—my body was beat, pooped, depleted. By that point, I was beginning to seriously dislike my practice—I was doing it more for her than me and didn't feel I could stop. I was counting the days until she left town—physically and mentally looking forward to taking a break so I wouldn't feel compelled to practice with this level of intensity, focus, drive. At the same time, I worried about keeping up my practice at all. I needed Priya's accountability, assistance, guidance, and encouragement. I told her I wasn't sure I could or would be able

PEACE, LOVE, AND YOGA

to maintain my practice while she was gone. "Just do your best," she said. "Take a break for a while, go to a few Vinyasa classes, and do a part of your practice each day if you can. You certainly don't have to do it all. Be kind to yourself and your body, Ellen. You'll be fine and we can pick back up when I return."

It didn't take long after she left for me to realize that I was in a mindset that wasn't healthy for me, one that recalled my triathlon mentality: *Push through the pain. Don't give up. Keep on going. You can't stop now.* When she left I felt a huge sense of relief, like, *Phew, I made it. And I've crossed the finish line.*

I went back to Vinyasa classes. I'd grown tired of the same Ashtanga sequence. It had become too repetitive, too routine, too structured. My head was too focused on the postures, and my heart yearned for a change. I wanted to think less and get lost in my practice, my breath, to connect all the eight limbs of yoga once again and free myself from my triathlon mentality. I embraced the fact that I had no idea what was coming next, no idea what the sequence was going to be. It was totally up to the instructor. It was freeing, and because of that, it was a much more joyful practice. Even if the sequence was less challenging one day, I took it as a sign from the Universe. That's exactly what my body needed today (to stay seated, to open my hips, to invert, or to stretch). I accepted that and approached each class with that mentality.

While Priya was away, we texted once or twice. I felt guilty about foregoing my practice and not doing what I was "supposed to be doing." I didn't want to let her down. Before departing for Mysore, Priya told me that she had decided to open her own *shala* in the home that she and her husband were building. I was thrilled for her.

211

I knew that was exactly what she wanted to do in order carry on the tradition of Ashtanga. She wanted to introduce others to the practice and create a space for those already connected to it to gather and grow their practice. But the area of town where she was building wasn't convenient for me at all. All of this started to sink in during our hiatus. I had also decided to become certified as a Lagree fitness instructor, completing the training during her time in Mysore. When I began teaching Lagree classes, my style was considerably influenced by the yoga instructors I admired—my expression was more authentic, focusing on students' form, breath, and strengthening the core, or *mula bandha*. I enjoyed teaching Lagree. The environment was much more intimate than the other gyms I had previously worked in. I loved training clients in a challenging, proven method that was new to Austin.

When Priya returned, we talked about her new shala and her opening schedule. Traditionally, a student of Ashtanga practices first thing in the morning on an empty stomach. She mentioned that she was planning on working her schedule around my availability. I told her I couldn't make afternoons because of my teaching schedule and that I couldn't make early morning because I had to drop a child at school. But Priya was more than willing to manage her schedule around mine. I had no excuse!

I took a deep breath and said, "I have to be honest with you. I am familiar with the rules of the shala. The requirement is that I practice a minimum of three days a week, though I can't commit to that right now. I totally respect how you choose to run your shala and want you to move forward, I just don't think I can be a part of it at this time. I think the break we took was meant for a reason." I told her I'd begun to resent the practice, that it was draining me, mentally and physically. It had become that monster I used to battle when I competed. I was putting too much pressure on myself to perform, to excel, to progress. I was getting lost in the postures and the true yoga was obscured by my desire to succeed. "The feeling is too familiar, Priya. I can't go there again."

I think she was stunned. I'd been so committed. I'd talked of studying the yoga sutras with her in her shala and traveling with her to Mysore. We talked through my decision, and although she accepted and respected it, I know she was hurt. But I don't regret the decision for a minute. I just have a hole in my heart where she once occupied space. I don't see Priya anymore, but I think about her all the time. She's a wonderful human being, I love what she's doing, but it's not right for me. The reason I embraced yoga was to be able to balance, ground, and get out of my head. I'd slipped back into that unhealthy space while practicing Ashtanga, but the good news was, I recognized the pattern and changed my course of action.

I was healing. Slowly, steadily. It's not that I didn't fall into old patterns again. I did, but I was now able to catch myself heading down an all-too-familiar path. I was paying attention to my body, noticing when I became too rigid, too obsessed with being perfect, too hard on myself, too busy, my temper short, my patience low, my thoughts racing—all signaling that I was stressed. By slowing down, easing up, taking a break from routine, I could get myself back on track.

It took effort. I thrived on chaos. I craved intensity. It was in my DNA. I realized that the adrenaline rush I got when I worked out, when I competed, was incredibly similar to the rush I got from being constantly busy, over-achieving, perpetually taking on more projects, more responsibility—I had to stay present to those impulses. And I was. Things were getting better.

Yoga still teaches me presence, compassion, and acceptance. I often feel self-conscious as I stare at my reflection in the mirrors in front of me. I see my imperfections, my misalignments, where I'm not balanced. Yoga can trigger the desire to one-up myself, to keep pushing, to do more, to get stronger, to hold a pose longer. There is always a pose or an inversion or an arm balance that I am striving to achieve or improve. Recognizing and accepting my strengths, and balancing them with self-compassion when the feeling of weakness arises, is the beauty of the yoga. As I begin to acknowledge these desires and cravings for more, I stop, breathe, and say to myself, *Oh, here you go again. Chill out, Ellen. Take a break. Peace, love, and yoga is all you need.*

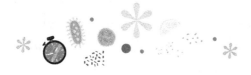

Epilogue

THE PATH HAS BEEN LONG, twisted, and challenging. I'm constantly reminding myself to stay present to my emotions and state of mind, to really pay attention to what is surfacing. The more comfortable I become with the feelings that arise when I'm stressed, tired, hungry, or angry, the easier I am able to navigate the forest through the trees. The path becomes clearer. I'm eternally watching myself. Self-awareness is key. As outfielder Leon Brown most eloquently said, "Listen to your own voice, your own soul. Too many people listen to the noise of the world, instead of themselves." Whether it's people or symptoms or the sound of your own breath, the answer is to connect—to one another and to ourselves. Keeping these relationships healthy and functioning at a high level is paramount to creating a better, more holistic life. I know how it feels to lose yourself. For so long, I disconnected from myself and I couldn't for the life of me find my way. The extraneous noise muffled my ability to trust my instincts. I've learned to be still and listen. To tune in to the beat of my heart, the melody of my soul, and the rhythm of my breath. That chorus makes my intuition sing. Take that shit and fertilize your truth. It will always lead you down the right path.

Now I'm able to listen from within and connect to *myself* like never before. I have a keen sense of awareness when something—my diet, my exercise, my health, the way I am feeling emotionally—is awry. Instead of second-guessing, disregarding the symptoms our bodies are sending, or just blowing hot air at the thoughts and feelings that come up, we need to call ourselves out and own that we're Full of Shit! I invite you to open your mind, connect to your innermost core, listen to your gut, and call your shit *your* shit. Get it together. The messages you receive are real. Pay attention to them, attend to them. You have the power to heal yourself. You have all the tools to cultivate your own health. As you gain clarity, truth will surface. Follow that intuition to eat, to rest, to reset, and flush all the rest down the toilet.

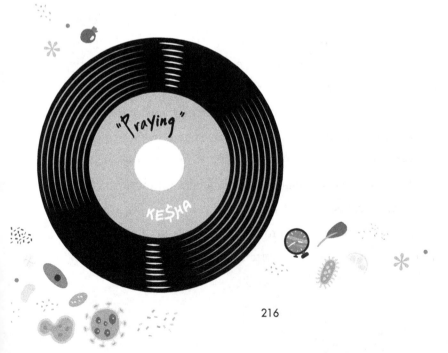

Acknowledgments

THIS BOOK HAS BEEN a labor of love, literally. Like a third child I haven't been able to birth. It's been in the womb, gestating, growing, developing for more than seven years. I could probably write another book mentioning all the people who've helped me deliver this baby, though I'll attempt to push it out in just a few short paragraphs.

To the grandparents, my mom and dad, Audrey and Charles, for conceiving me and for not throwing their baby out with the bathwater. I know it was tempting at times! I love you!

Kelly Malone, you're incredible. You held my hand and told me I could do this. Your knowledge, expertise, and friendship have been my guiding light. You are the doula of all the details.

Blythe Jewell, Jaclyn Hubersberger, Nettie Reynolds, Katherine Moore—my neonatal nurses who assisted me through the incubation phase while I was trying to write this book.

Rosa Schnyer, Kerry Meath-Sinkin, Priya Jhawar, Mark Herbert, Daniel Kalish, Chris Kresser, Gerard Mullin—my nurse practitioners who gave me advice and support, and from whom I learned so much along the way (point of clarification, some of the aforementioned are real medical docs).

Dr. Michael Lindstrom, thank you. Without you there would be no story to tell.

Dr. Mark Dickey, your prescription put me on the path back to health, where I was actually able to conceive and create.

Bianca Krause, Maria Orozova, Stefanie Rubenfield, and The MOD Studio for putting a face with a name. You truly brought life to this book with your beautiful illustrations and creative eye.

Stephanie Smith and Genie Leslie, my lactation consultants, who helped me nourish this baby by making sure all of my "t's" were crossed and my "i's" were dotted before we went to print.

Marisa Jackson, your creativity and eye for design created the layette for this baby, making sure it was covered from head to toe and dressed for success.

Rashana Moss and Shannon Pike, for helping this baby find her muse.

Lynn Yeldell, you got this baby on the web and created a social media presence for her because every kid needs an Instagram account!

Cecily Sailer, the fairy-godmother whose multi-faceted magic provided this nervous new parent the final set of eyes I needed before taking this baby to print.

The Universe, for showing me the way, always and forever.

About the Author

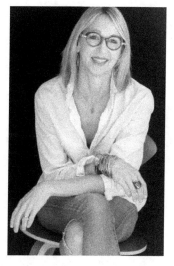

ELLEN ROZMAN is a connector of foodies, farmers, fitness enthusiasts, and functional medicine followers. She has a fetish for eyeglass frames and is maladroit at managing social media.

As The Locavore Next Door, Ellen is constantly connecting community to local food, local farms, and local businesses. She is incessantly interested in the microbiome and geeks out about the gut-brain connection. While no longer twenty-something, for that many years she's enjoyed educating people by focusing on fitness and food to further improve their health.

Her passion for seasonal sustainable food and community-centered wellness progressed as her personal challenges with food and fitness peaked.

Ellen calls Austin, Texas, her home. She lives with her husband, Mark; daughter, Shaine; son, Harrison; and mini-golden doodle, Karma. Get in touch to book a gig, reach out about a reading, or just drop a line to lend some love or share some shit.

Learn more about the book and related events at fullofshitbook.com.
Send email to ellen@fullofshitbook.com.

CPSIA information can be obtained
at www.ICGtesting.com
Printed in the USA
LVHW081114040323
740904LV00002B/45

9 780999 743904